*Get Through*

**The Foundation Years:
A Handbook for Junior
Doctors**

# *Get Through*

# The Foundation Years: A Handbook for Junior Doctors

*Editor*

Ashis Banerjee FRCS FFAEM
Consultant in Emergency Medicine
University Hospital, Lewisham, London, UK

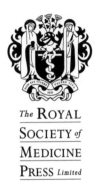

*The* ROYAL
SOCIETY *of*
MEDICINE
PRESS *Limited*

© 2005 Royal Society of Medicine Press Ltd
Published by the Royal Society of Medicine Press Ltd
1 Wimpole Street, London W1G 0AE, UK
Tel: +44 (0)20 7290 2921
Fax: +44 (0)20 7290 2929
Email: *publishing@rsm.ac.uk*
Website: *www.rsmpress.co.uk*

**British Library Cataloguing in Publication Data**
A catalogue record for this book is available from the British Library

ISBN 1-85315-691-4

Distribution in Europe and Rest of World:
Marston Book Services Ltd
PO Box 269
Abingdon
Oxon OX14 4YN, UK
Tel: +44 (0)1235 465500
Fax: +44 (0)1235 465555
Email: *direct.order@marston.co.uk*

Distribution in the USA and Canada:
Royal Society of Medicine Press Ltd
c/o Jamco Distribution Inc
1401 Lakeway Drive
Lewisville, TX 75057, USA
Tel: +1 800 538 1287
Fax: +1 972 353 1303
Email: *jamco@majors.com*

Distribution in Australia and New Zealand:
Elsevier Australia
30–52 Smidmore Street, Marrikville NSW 2204, Australia
Tel: +61 2 9517 8999
Fax: +61 2 9517 2249
Email: *service@elsevier.com.au*

Typeset by Phoenix Photosetting, Chatham, Kent
Printed in the UK by Bell & Bain Ltd, Glasgow

# Contents

# Preface

Postgraduate medical education is in a period of reorganization and resultant turmoil and junior doctors embarking on foundation year training may reasonably feel uncertain about their career progression. This book has been written with the aim of helping to resolve current uncertainties, while also providing useful information on a variety of issues relating to the restructuring.

The contributors come from a wide range of backgrounds, in terms of both vintage and perspective, and have come together to produce a book which, it is hoped, will be of considerable help to junior doctors. Feedback would be most welcome as well as suggestions for additions to the text that might be included in future editions.

AB

# List of contributors

**Romila Bahl** BSc(Hons), MBBS, MRCP, Specialist Registrar in Emergency Medicine, Queen Elizabeth Hospital, Woolwich

**Ashis Banerjee** FRCS, FFAEM, Consultant in Emergency Medicine, University Hospital, Lewisham

**Simon Edward** MBBS, Senior House Officer in Emergency Medicine, University Hospital, Lewisham

**Vijay Hajela** MRCP, Consultant Rheumatologist, University Hospital, Lewisham

**Nigel Harrison** FRCS, FFAEM, Consultant in Emergency Medicine, University Hospital, Lewisham

**Gordon Jackson** FRCP, Consultant Cardiologist, University Hospital, Lewisham, and Site-Dean, GKT School of Medicine, Lewisham Campus

**Louise Ma** MBBS, Foundation Year 2 Senior House Officer in Care of the Elderly, University Hospital, Lewisham

**Girish Malde** MBBS, FRCS, MSc, MRCGP, general practitioner; trainer and course organizer, Lewisham VTS

**Giles Walker** MRCP, Associate Specialist, Gastroenterology, University Hospital, Lewisham

# 1 Modernizing medical careers

**Romila Bahl**

Modernizing Medical Careers (MMC) has a broad remit and deciphering its intention can be confusing. Phrases such as 'competency-based', 'seamless transition' and 'run-through training' have made their way into everyday medical dialect. However, working out what this means for doctors in training can be overwhelming. This chapter defines some of these terms, explores the background to MMC, examines the relevant papers and offers a 'Who's Who' of the significant organizations. It will give an overview of the new careers pathway, what the Royal Colleges and Junior Doctors Committee (JDC) currently think, and answer some common concerns. MMC is not just about Foundation programmes; it involves every aspect of a doctor's career. Things are rapidly changing and so being informed is essential.

## What is MMC?

MMC is a radical rethink of postgraduate medical training, based on many factors that impart upon and integrate with one another. The essential concerns being addressed are as follows.

- What do patients want and require?
- What is the best way that training can be structured in order to produce a workforce with the skills required for the modernized NHS?
- How long does it take to train a doctor without compromising standards?
- Is it necessary for all doctors to be as specialized as they are currently?
- What skills must a doctor demonstrate in order to progress in training?
- What are the needs of doctors in training?

# Why MMC?

In *The NHS Plan*, published July 2000, the government recognized that a reform of doctors' training was required and in *A Health Service for All the Talents* (February 2001), it made a commitment to review the Senior House Officer (SHO) grade. The Registrar grade had undergone significant restructuring after the Calman Report published in 1993. Although this improved higher specialist training (HST), problems existed in both basic training and the routes of entry to HST. The over-riding government concern was a need for better systems of care for patients. Its commitment to changing junior doctor training was cemented in March 2005 by £73 million of funding.

## The SHO perspective: *Unfinished Business*[1]

Compiled in August 2002 by the Chief Medical Officer Sir Liam Donaldson, this report reviewed the need for change at SHO grade. Half the doctors in the UK at that time were employed as SHOs, one-third of these being non-UK graduates. These posts had a disproportionate slant to service and lacked cohesion in their training, leading to the now often quoted terms 'workhorses of the NHS' and 'lost tribe'. There was recognition of the bottleneck that existed as doctors tried to enter specialist training and also the variability of career progression at SHO level, problems compounded by the increasing numbers of 'trust grade' posts being created to meet service demand. The report highlighted the principles of SHO training reform: 'Time limited, broadly based programmes, accountable and structured, closely managed and flexible for the individual'.

## The changing needs of the NHS: tailoring training to requirements

There has been an imbalance between need and the number of doctors applying for certain specialties, resulting in too many doctors wanting to practise in one area and not enough in another. There have even been cases of doctors at the end of their specialist training not having consultant jobs to go to. As well as problems with the simple logistics of workforce planning, there has been a growing feeling that the NHS needed more trained generalists to provide safe and effective patient care. There is a desire for a service delivered by trained doctors, rather than trainees. MMC recognizes that the NHS is changing, with new working patterns such as Hospital at Night, European Working Time Directive requirements and an increasing awareness of the patient's perspective.

## The need for increasing accountability

A number of high-profile cases and growing public awareness of health provision meant that there was pressure for clearer accountability of the training process, with doctors achieving a predefined set of competencies before being able to progress. Patients wanted clarity of what to expect from doctors below the grade of consultant or GP.

## European Union law

The European Economic Area agreement ('Freedom of Movement of Goods, People, Services and Capital, January 2004), along with a concurrent widening of the European Economic Area, meant that postgraduate medical education needed to adapt to this diverse single market. 'Non-UK trained doctors should have their needs fairly taken into account and have fair access to jobs in line with EU legislation'.[2]

## The current documents in MMC

*Modernizing Medical Careers – The Next Steps* (April 2004)[3]

This policy document states: 'The MMC initiative takes a radical look at the way we train doctors, the speed and quality with which we do it and the end product of that process. It examines the opportunities for streamlining training and increasing flexibility, a move to competency-based training throughout the medical continuum'. This document defined the standards for Foundation programme training and detailed programme structure. It defined the new career pathway of 'seamless transition' from medical school to Foundation programme to higher specialist training and, subject to satisfactory progress against defined assessments, a Certificate of Completion of Training (CCT). It also detailed the timeline for Foundation programmes starting in August 2005.

*Choice and Opportunity Proposals for Modernizing Non-Consultant Career Grades* (July 2003)[4]

This document examined the role of non-consultant career grades and suggested a new career structure with competency-based assessment for entry and progression, also as a means to gain entry to Specialist Registrar (SpR) training if desired.

*Modernizing Medical Careers – Response of Four UK Health Departments to 'Unfinished Business'* (February 2003)[5]

This is a policy statement from the four UK health departments detailing key principles for postgraduate medical education reform in response to the consultation process that happened after the publication of *Unfinished Business*. It also outlined some of the work required to happen.

*The Shape of Specialist Training: Aspirations for Seamless Progression* (JDC 2005)[6]

This document gave suggestions for pathways from the Foundation programme into specialist training and the criteria required by junior doctors from the new training programmes – flexibility, careers counselling, numbered progression, opportunities for all who complete a Foundation programme to enter a specialty training programme in a seamless manner, rigorous in-training assessment, competency-based assessment not time-based progression.

*The New Doctor – Recommendations on General Clinical Training* (GMC January 2005)[7]

This document details the outcomes that Pre-Registration House Officers (PRHOs) must show they have achieved before full registration is granted. It aims to be fully implemented at the end of August 2007.

## Who's who in MMC

*Postgraduate Medical Education and Training Board* (PMETB)

This board was established by legislation in April 2003, started work in October 2003 and is independent of the government. Its 'Go Live' date is

September 2005 when it will start to take over its new responsibilities using the systems currently in place alongside new requirements. Its wider aims are: modernization, professional self-regulation and connection of the institutes of postgraduate medical education with more involvement of the public and patients. The PMETB hopes to bring consistency and integration, being the one organization with collective responsibility for postgraduate medical education and being accountable for ensuring that the standards it sets are met. It will work with the Royal Colleges and deaneries and take over the Specialist Training Authority's (STA) role of the regulation and awarding of Certificates of Completion of Specialist Training (CCST). To date, the board has independently reviewed the 73 curricula involved in postgraduate medical education and is due to discuss these with the Royal Colleges. It will have ultimate responsibility for these curricula. From July 2005 it has been developing the vision for its future and hopes to roll out new procedures and systems from January 2006.

## The GMC

The GMC is the profession's regulating body, concerned with the protection of patients and maintaining the standards the public have a right to expect. It will still be responsible for the registration of all new doctors, setting the standards for what needs to have been achieved before full registration and the quality assurance of undergraduate education. Progress in year 1 of the Foundation programme will be the responsibility of the GMC and PMETB. There had been debate on whether full registration could be made earlier than the end of Foundation year 1 but EU legislation requires six years or 5500 hours of theoretical and practical instruction supervised by a university for registration.

## The deaneries

The deaneries are responsible for the delivery of postgraduate medical education to doctors in training. Most have application packs on their websites for Foundation programmes in their region.

## The Royal Colleges and faculties

The Royal Colleges are currently responsible for setting the standards of entry to their specialty, the curriculum for specialty training and criteria for examinations. This role will become part of the remit of the PMETB, though it is likely that the Colleges will act either as agents of the PMETB or in close conjunction.

## The MMC Group

This is the UK strategy group set up to develop the thinking and principles of MMC. It is headed by Sir Liam Donaldson and involves members from the following bodies:

- GMC
- Royal Colleges
- JCPTGP
- Specialist Training Authority of medical colleges (STA)
- PMTEB
- Conference of Postgraduate Medical Education Deans (CoPMED)
- Committee of GP Education Directors (CoGPED).

It prepared the *Next Steps* document and more recently made a number of decisions on the curriculum and assessment tools to be used in the Foundation years.

## MMC Working Party

This is the group responsible for overseeing change. It is currently involved in piloting assessment tools and working with the GMC and PMETB to ensure that Foundation programmes start on time in August 2005. Its website is a useful source of information about what has happened and what is planned.

The current implementation schedule

- 31 March 2005 Foundation programme curriculum out
- April 2005 Purple guide (operational framework for FP) – similar to the orange guide to SpR training
- May 2005 Rough guide to the Foundation programme
- June 2005 Selection methods for specialist training agreed in principle
- June 2005 Foundation programme begins
- August 2005 SAS grade restructuring plan agreed
- September 2005 Specialty Review conclusions
- October 2005 Workforce transition management arrangements agreed
- August 2006 Application process for specialty selection agreed
- August 2007 First MMC cohort enters specialist training

# The new careers pathway

MMC will mean a new careers pathway for doctors. The stages involved are as follows.

## Medical school

More careers guidance. Students should consider what they eventually want to do and tailor some areas of choice within the curriculum to their areas of interest. Such areas could include electives, a special study module, intercalated BSc course and prizes.

## Foundation programme: years 1 and 2

This is covered in Chapter 2 but briefly involves:

- matching by medical schools and the deaneries into UK-wide, two-year Foundation programmes
- programmes to be standardized and offer exposure to acute medicine and surgery with some choice for other areas.

## Selection to higher specialist training

This is an area of much debate and will be discussed in more detail below. The aims of *The Next Steps* are 'open competition, midway in Foundation year 2, for selection into higher specialist training'. This competition will provide equal access for non-UK graduates. There should be no further competition and prior experience should not be a selection criterion.

## Progress: higher specialist training

Once on a higher specialist programme, the trainee should be secure in their career pathway if progress is satisfactory with respect to explicit outcomes. The programmes should be sufficiently flexible to allow for time out, movement to other areas or a switch to non-consultant grades if preferred. Career choice should be matched with NHS requirements. Programmes will vary from two to six years, depending on specialty, and result in the award of a Certificate of Completion of Training (CCT). There is debate about what happens for specialty training within the broad areas. For example, if someone wants to be a respiratory physician, do they train for this period in respiratory medicine only, do they pursue both internal and respiratory medicine, as is the current pattern, or do they train beyond CCT in their chosen subspecialty? The role for the Royal College examinations as part of the HST process is also being debated.

## Exit: beyond CCT or CCST

The consultant may be a generalist or may wish to undertake postspecialization training or carry out research. There is currently no decision as to selection processes and cost implications for post-CCT training. Also, in order to be listed by the large private insurance companies, a doctor needs to be on the specialist register or equivalent. Whether the award of a CCT will be the equivalent of a CCST remains to be seen and may indeed vary with specialty.

# Selection criteria for higher specialist training: when and what?

There is a general feeling that making a final career choice once and for all 18 months after leaving medical school could be problematic; one-third of doctors have no clear focused intention at that point. There is also the question of what selection criteria should be used for open competition. The Foundation programme assessments are generic, not examination or specialty based. Determining aptitude or interest on these alone may not be realistic. Currently selection into many areas of higher specialist training is based on basic specialty experience and passing membership examinations. This does not fit in with the principles outlined in *The Next Steps*.

## Suggestions from the JDC

The basic idea of the JDC is a one-point selection at entry to specialist training. Whatever training is undertaken should count towards final accreditation; there should be flexibility and the opportunity to change careers. The way the selection would work would be dependent on the individual's confidence in their career choice and structure of specialist training in their chosen field. Possible career progression could be as follows.

- *Certain of what you want to do*: competitive entry midway through FY2 to a numbered specialist post or GP training. Follow the programme and progress via defined competencies. Programmes should still have exposure to general areas if applicable.
- *Unsure*: choose to do a broader based programme, for example acute care. This may involve ITU, anaesthetics, A&E, acute medicine and other related areas. The additional experience and career guidance would then lead to entry to specialist training with the time in this broader programme counting towards CCT. Time spend in a broader based programme should not be used as a general selection criterion for specialist training.

It is anticipated that the first year of specialist training would contain generic medical skills and would be similar across specialties, making it easier to incorporate time spent and experience as credits to HST. The timing of competitive entry to final specialist training would need flexibility to allow the broader based programmes to run in parallel with the direct entry after the Foundation years.

## What the Colleges think about selection

Website details are given at the end of the chapter for further information. Follow the links to 'a career in' and keep up to date in your area of interest. Things are likely to change as decisions are made and refined.

### Royal College of Surgeons

Quoting from Bernard Ribeiro, Vice President, Royal College of Surgeons of England: 'Some surgical specialties will be shorter than others, varying from five to eight years post Foundation programme'. The College would like a portfolio of interests and skills to determine selection into the first year of surgical training and then further assessment of skills and knowledge and competitive entry to determine entry to the rest of specialist training, with opportunities for competitive entry for doctors from abroad, research or changing careers at appropriate stages. If the specialty is suited, there could also be 'fast-tracking' from the Foundation years to specialist training.

### Royal College of Physicians

The priorities as stated by Dr George Cowan, Medical Director of the Joint Committee of Higher Medical Training (JCHMT), are: 'All physicians need adequate training in general medicine, with time for MRCP and career choice' and 'The NHS requires not general physicians but acute medical physicians, specialists both in internal medicine and the broad specialties, mono-specialists and also academics'.

The proposed basic template is similar to the current process with appropriate alterations when the end career is in a mono-specialty.

### Royal College of Anaesthetists

Dr Peter Simpson, President of the Royal College of Anaesthetists, states that 'The specialty already has competency-based assessments with exams integral to this as part of specialist training'. There could be competitive entry to specialist training either directly from the Foundation programme or from a common acute/critical care stem. Competitive entry could include consideration of academic record at medical school (including a relevant BSc) and the relevant FY1 and 2 competencies.

## Royal College of Psychiatrists

Dr Gareth Holsgrove, Medical Advisor to the Royal College of Psychiatrists, feels that selection criteria to higher training after FY2 will be very important. The College is already involved in devising the new curriculum for specialist training based on GMC requirements for *Good Medical Practice*. Access to modules of HST could be on offer to non-psychiatrists for continuing professional development (CPD).

## Royal College of Paediatrics and Child Health

The College has stated a desire to maintain the role of the College examination for progression and also to maintain flexibility in its specialist training. By the nature of the specialty, it is felt that paediatricians need to recognize both the rare and common and need expertise in a wide range of specialties.

## Royal College of Obstetricians and Gynaecologists

The College's position, as stated by President Professor Allan Templeton, is 'Training time should not be shortened. Trainees would have three years of core specialist training equipping them to deal with most emergencies and obstetric situations, then undergo two years of special skills training, with the option of a further year for subspecialization'. The possibility of a transition year after the Foundation programme has been suggested.

## Royal College of General Practitioners

The information sheet produced in February 2005, available on their website, is very informative.

The College has advised that all doctors should experience general practice as part of their Foundation years. Then there should be open competition to a three-year HST programme for those wishing to pursue a career in general practice. After successful completion of HST, the doctor will be able to apply for career-grade GP posts. The College is continuing to push for higher professional education in the early years after CCT.

Royal College of Radiologists

Previously entry followed a College exam such as MRCP or MRCS. With MMC, the emphasis will change to other means of assessing interest and enthusiasm. The College suggests that the guidelines may well alter but currently advises showing an interest in radiology with relevant audit or research projects or electives, fostering links with your local department and attending relevant meetings and keeping a portfolio of imaging-related projects.

Royal College of Pathologists

The College has drafted a document for 'run-through' training in histopathology to be pioneered in August 2005.

# Common questions

## *I'm on a Foundation programme: what does it mean for me?*

From August 2005 graduates will start on two-year Foundation programmes. Midway in FY2 it is envisaged that there will be a selection process for specialist training, the criteria for selection to specialist training was agreed in principle by June 2005 and the application process for specialty selection to be agreed in August 2006. This means that there will be six months between the agreement of the process and the first doctors going through it. Keep informed of what the process is going to be and bear in mind the the competencies taken as part of the Foundation year are likely to have a role. MMC and the PMETB have stated competition will be open, which means that selection criteria should be explicit and clear. Find out what they are as soon as they are published by the PMETB, MMC and Colleges in June 2005 and let this inform any decisions.

## *What if my Foundation programme does not include the specialty I'm interested in?*

Don't panic if the Foundation programme you are on does not include your intended specialty. It has been stated by the PMETB that this should not be a consideration for selection into specialty training. If you know what you want to do, find out about the specialty via relevant websites and make sure this is an informed choice. Discuss it with your consultants and those currently in the specialty. Think about how your profile shows that you are interested in that specialty.

## I'm currently an SHO. Where will I fit in?

There will inevitably be some 'bumps' as the new system is introduced. To minimize disruption to your career plan, it is worth working out where it is you want to work, in what area and where you currently stand with respect to experience so far. Then take careers advice and follow the College careers pathways, keeping up to date with proposed changes.

There may need to be a process of equivalence for those entering higher specialist training directly from Foundation programmes and those who entered already with basic specialist training so have a list of how much you have already done. You'll need it anyway for your CC(S)T or vocational training post.

## Do I take the College exams?

The membership exams are supported by most of the Colleges as appropriate to specialist training. Their current role as part of the selection criteria for entry to specialist training may change. At the time of writing, it is envisaged that the new selection criteria will apply from August 2007. All the Colleges publish career pathways on their websites and most of these include taking the membership exams and obtaining basic specialist experience as an SHO.

## What about going abroad?

Going abroad between Foundation years may cause some logistic headaches so consider when it would be best to go and take advice from your mentors on this. If you want your time abroad to count towards training, make sure the post is recognized for training by the appropriate College of the country you are visiting before you go and get documentation of your satisfactory completion of the job at the end. If you want to travel/do voluntary work/half-work, half-fun, then do so but keep a list of what you do. It's all part of your profile and you may be surprised at when it could come in useful. If you know what you want to do when you return, then research this before you go and take advice from your intended area.

## What if I just don't know?

Don't panic! Talk to your consultants, take stock of what you like doing and where you see yourself in a few years' time. Find out about the end point of training in the specialties that may interest you and most of all, keep informed. Each trust will have a Foundation Programme Director who can point you in the right direction for advice. MMC is meant to be flexible and it is intended that credits for time in different related areas will count to specialist training. Keep informed about the broader career choices that may be available.

# References

1. Donaldson L. *Unfinished Business: Proposals for the Reform of the Senior House Officer Grade. A Paper for Consultation*. London: Stationery Office, 2002.
2. Postgraduate Medical Education and Training Board. *PMETB – The First Three Years*. London: PMETB, 2004.
3. Department of Health, Social Services and Public Safety, Scottish Executive, Welsh Assembly Government. *Modernizing Medical Careers – The Next Steps. The Future Shape of Foundation, Specialist and General Practice Training Programmes*. London: Department of Health, 2003.
4. Department of Health. *Choice and Opportunity – Proposals for Modernizing Non-Consultant Career Grades*. London: Department of Health, 2003.
5. Department of Health, Social Services and Public Safety, Scottish Executive, Welsh Assembly Government. *Modernizing Medical Careers – Response of the Four UK Health Departments to 'Unfinished Business'*. London: Department of Health, 2003.
6. BMA Junior Doctors Committee. *The Shape of Specialist Training: Aspirations for Seamless Progression*. London: British Medical Association, 2005.
7. General Medical Council. *The New Doctor – Recommendations on General Clinical Training*. London: General Medical Council, 2005.

# Useful websites

*www.mmc.nhs.uk* The website for up-to-date information on the MMC project. Also provides links to all the deaneries, MMC newsletters, a frequently asked questions section and the option of emailing the MMC team with any queries.

*www.pmetb.org.uk/pmetb* The home of the Postgraduate Medical Education and Training Board. Contains all the PMETB publications, news and updates and information about curricula and certification.

*www.bmjcareers.com* Gives access to an online version of Career Focus, the BMJ's weekly supplement. There is also an archive of previous issues.

*www.dh.gov.uk* The website for the Department of Health in England – very useful for keeping up to date with government health initiatives and for finding publications of policy.

*www.gmc-uk.org* The website of the General Medical Council.

The Royal Colleges:
*www.rcseng.ac.uk* Royal College of Surgeons of England
*www.rcplondon.ac.uk* Royal College of Physicians
*www.rcoa.ac.uk* Royal College of Anaesthetists
*www.rcpsych.ac.uk* Royal College of Psychiatrists
*www.rcpch.ac.uk* Royal College of Paediatrics and Child Health
*www.rcog.org.uk* Royal College of Obstetricians and Gynaecologists
*www.rcgp.org.uk* Royal College of General Practitioners
*www.rcr.ac.uk* Royal College of Radiologists
*www.rcpath.org* Royal College of Pathologists
*www.faem.org.uk* Faculty of Accident and Emergency Medicine

# 2

# Foundation training in the UK

Vijay Hajela

## What is a Foundation programme?

A Foundation programme is a two-year period of postgraduate medical training designed to provide newly qualified doctors with a sound platform in clinical practice. The first Foundation programmes will start in August 2005. The first year will equate to the current Pre-registration House Officer (PRHO) year. The second year will be a generic first year of SHO training. Each two-year programme will be made up of a series of placements with educational links between them. As with PRHO training, GMC registration would be expected at the end of the first year of Foundation training. A particular emphasis for Foundation programme trainees will be the recognition and management of acutely sick patients. Progress through the two years will be determined by a series of work-based assessments of clinical competence. The first year of Foundation programme training is sometimes referred to as the F1 year and the second year as the F2 year.

## The need for change: *Unfinished Business*[1] and *Modernizing Medical Careers*[2]

Half of all doctors in training are SHOs yet for a long time there have been concerns about SHO training. In 2002 the Chief Medical Officer published a paper entitled *Unfinished Business: Reform of the Senior House Officer Grade*. It concluded that current SHO training:

- is poorly planned; half of all SHO jobs are short term and not part of any structured rotation

- is too long; in many cases doctors spend 4–6 years as an SHO before managing to move onto specialty or GP training
- is inadequately supervised, with poorly informed appraisal
- fails to take into account the training requirements of non-UK graduates (one-third of SHOs are non-UK graduates)
- has inadequate selection and appointment procedures.

A subsequent consultation exercise resulted in the proposal for a radical overhaul of junior doctor training. This reform of postgraduate medical training, known as Modernizing Medical Careers, was launched in February 2003. The Foundation programme will be the first phase of Modernizing Medical Careers to be implemented.

Patient safety is currently high on the political agenda. Central to this is the need for doctors to demonstrate that they are competent to do the job required of them in a modern National Health Service. This is one of the major objectives of Modernizing Medical Careers, hence the Foundation programme.

## Timescale for implementing Foundation training

The first cohort of F1 trainees will start in August 2005. In August 2006, the first year of F2 training will begin. The proposed 'run-through' grade will commence the following year in 2007.

- F1 year starts August 2005
- F2 year starts August 2006
- 'Run-through grade' starts August 2007

## The aims of Foundation training

The key aims of Foundation training are for newly qualified doctors to:

- develop the generic personal, professional and clinical skills required to be a good doctor
- experience a wide range of medical practice in different settings
- demonstrate fitness for full GMC registration
- make well-informed career choices.

## Responsibility for overseeing Foundation programmes

Whilst the GMC will remain responsible for overseeing the F1 year, a new body called the Postgraduate Medical Education and Training Board

(PMETB) will be responsible for the approval and quality assurance of the F2 year. Deaneries will be responsible for implementing and managing the programmes.

## Foundation schools

Foundation schools will be a partnership between undergraduate medical schools and postgraduate deans in order to help them manage the large number of placements which together will form F1 and F2 programmes. Each Foundation school will offer placements in acute trusts, general practice, mental health trusts and other suitable settings. Recruitment to Foundation programmes will be made through Foundation schools.

## Entry to Foundation programmes

Most graduates from UK medical schools will gain entry to Foundation programmes by applying to the Foundation school linked to their medical school. If a graduate wants to apply to a Foundation school in another part of the country then they will need to seek permission from their own university beforehand (according to GMC regulations).

It is thought that most Foundation schools will only allocate graduates to the F1 year initially. The allocation of F2 placements will be managed by postgraduate deans and is likely to take place 6–9 months through the F1 year. The exact way in which this allocation will take place is still uncertain.

For non-UK graduates the requirement for entry to Foundation programmes is likely to be the successful completion of both PRHO posts and PLAB (Professional and Linguistic Assessment Board) tests. They will enter Foundation programmes at the F2 level, competing in an open and standardized application process.

## The structure and content of Foundation programmes

The duration of placements within Foundation programmes will vary. Around the country there will be programmes with $4 \times 3$ months, $3 \times 4$ months and $2 \times 6$ months jobs within both F1 and F2 years. It is expected that over 50% of Foundation programmes will eventually offer experience in primary care, although this may be difficult to achieve initially.

F1 rotations will consist mainly of medicine and surgery posts, like the current PRHO year. This is because three months of both medicine and surgery are required for full GMC registration.

F2 years will vary greatly. Some will be themed for those who are keen to get surgical or medical experience. Many will offer a variety of experience. Most trainees will have A&E as part of their F2 programme.

## How Foundation training will differ from what happens now

Foundation programmes will be more structured and trainee centred than traditional PRHO and SHO training. There will be a greater emphasis on the achievement of generic skills, e.g. team working and the management of acutely sick patients. Other key features are outlined below.

### Curriculum

A curriculum has been produced for the Foundation years of postgraduate medical training.[3] No such curriculum used to exist for PRHO or SHO training.

### Portfolio

Each trainee will have a training portfolio. It will be used to record their training objectives and to keep the results of assessments, presentations and other activities. This will provide a body of evidence to help demonstrate their competence in various domains of medical practice. It will provide a focus for discussion at their subsequent appraisals and help with producing a personal development plan. Work is ongoing to produce an electronic version of the training portfolio but this is unlikely to be ready for August 2005.

### Assessment of competencies

Each trainee will undergo a series of in-work assessments in both F1 and F2 years. These assessments will be used to gauge a trainee's clinical and personal skills, e.g. history taking and examination, how well they communicate with patients and other members of the multidisciplinary team and how competently they can perform basic medical procedures. Another important feature of all assessments is the immediate feedback of a trainee's performance by the senior colleague who supervises the assessment. Assessment in Foundation programmes is discussed in much more detail in Chapter 7.

## Wider experience

Shorter placements will allow trainees to gain experience of a wider range of specialties. In addition, many programmes will allow trainees to gain additional experience particularly in minority specialties. Several schemes have been piloted, including week-long 'taster' programmes and half-day releases in primary care.

## Concerns

Despite the anticipated benefits of Foundation training, there are several concerns.

- The conflict between service provision and the educational needs of trainees is likely to be greater than ever before.
- How to train the large number of personnel (medical and allied healthcare professionals) required for competency assessments
- Will Foundation schools be ready to cope with the enormous task of allocating places to both F1 and F2 years?
- What happens after F2? There seems to be considerable confusion about how run-through training will work in different specialties.

# References

1. Donaldson L. *Unfinished Business*: *Proposals for Reform of the Senior House Officer Grade*. London: Stationery Office, 2002.
2. Department of Health, Social Services and Public Safety, Scottish Executive, Welsh Assembly Government. *Modernizing Medical Careers – Response of the Four UK Health Departments to 'Unfinished Business'*. London: Department of Health, 2003.
3. Academy of Medical Royal Colleges and MMC Implementation Groups of the Department of Health, Scottish Executive and Welsh Assembly. *Curriculum for the Foundation Years in Postgraduate Education and Training*. London: Department of Health, 2005.

# Useful websites

*www.mmc.nhs.uk* Modernizing Medical Careers website: very useful source of information and good links to other sites of interest.

*www.gmc-uk.org* General Medical Council website with information about *The New Doctor* (Jan 2005). This sets out the learning objectives for the first year of Foundation training.

*www.dh.gov.uk* For details of *Unfinished Business: Proposals for Reform of the Senior House Officer Grade.*

*www.dh.gov.uk/PublicationsAndStatistics/Publications/PublicationsLibrary* For details of important publications by the Chief Medical Officer.

# 3

# What to look for in F2 programmes and beyond

**Gordon Jackson**

It is appropriate to begin this chapter with a health warning. In writing it, I have to make it quite clear that I do not know what one should be looking for in an F2 programme and I have no idea what lies beyond. My experience of the change in medical training that goes by the name of Modernizing Medical Careers is that, thus far, it has been long on rhetoric and particularly short on detail.

One of the ironies of the situation is that the rhetoric tells us that the Foundation years should be a time when newly qualified doctors are better able to plan their career based on better advice and experience than ever before. I know that as someone working in a hospital where we have tried to provide the best possible career support to pre-registration housemen for the last 15 years, I now find myself unable to give much in the way of useful advice and in the case of final-year students entering the Foundation year in August 2005, I find myself quite unable to give any useful advice at all.

---

**Box 3.1  What we know about the F2 year**

It is due to start in August 2006.

- Pilot schemes are currently in progress and it should be possible to gain some information from them before August 2006.
- The F2 year will be a single entity. That is, holders of an F2 post or rotation can expect to spend the year in the same trust or in the community related to that trust.
- Full registration with the GMC will occur after the first year of medical practice, as it does now. An F1 trainee will be a pre-registration doctor as now and an F2 trainee will be a registered doctor.
- Most F2 years will consist of a series of short rotations of two, three or four months.

---

---

**Box 3.2   What we do not know about the F2 year**

- The mechanism of appointment to the year. Will graduation from a UK medical school ensure automatic progression from F1 to F2 (given satisfactory completion of F1)?
- The mix of specialties which a typical rotation will contain.

---

## Some likely features of the F2 year

- It seems likely that admission to F2 training will be by competitive entry. Obviously if this is truly competitive with no safety net, then we know that satisfactory completion of the F1 year cannot guarantee entry to F2.
- It seems likely that some sort of national template for admission to the F2 year will be developed and that this will be used on a regional (deanery) basis.
- It seems likely that if College professional exams (MRCP, MRCS, etc.) remain essential for entry into higher specialist training, it will not be possible to take them until after the F2 year.

## What might a typical F2 programme contain?

The development of competence in the management of acutely ill patients is one of the points emphasized in the rhetoric supporting the change to Foundation programmes. It follows from this that over the course of a two-year period, there is likely to be substantial experience in A&E and related areas such as acute medical admission units. It seems likely that this period (or these periods) will be in the F2 part of the programme. Thus the service needs of the NHS and the stated intention of promoting competence in the care of acutely ill patients will lead to most F2 rotations having a substantial proportion of A&E in them.

If we take the F1 and F2 years together it seems that there are a number of pieces that have to be in the jigsaw. In order to register, pre-registration doctors must have performed their requisite periods of at least three months in surgery and three months in medicine. The remaining six months as a PRHO can be spent in any recognized clinical specialty or specialties. In reality, the majority of pre-registration years are made up of two six-month periods (or $2 \times 3$ months in medicine and $2 \times 3$ months in surgery) with a substantial minority made up of three four-month periods. This may change over time but as the first F1 programmes come into being in August 2005, it seems highly likely that there will be little change in the basic rotations from the previous PRHO programme (the process of assessment, appraisal and so on will have to change to fit in with the requirements of the F1 year). From this it follows that for most, general practice experience, if it takes place at all, will have to wait until the F2 year.

In March 2005, John Hutton, a Minister of Health, announced an additional £73 million to support the funding of the Foundation programme. It seems clear from the information accompanying the press release on this additional funding that much will be devoted to funding placements in general practice for the Foundation years. It is a stated intention that most people completing their Foundation programme will have had experience of general practice. There are, of course, many examples of PRHO rotations that contain general practice and it is likely that some GP elements of Foundation training will take place in the F1 year whilst others take place in the F2 year. However, if we accept that periods in A&E and primary care are a likely part of the majority of F2 programmes, it follows that for a substantial proportion of F2 postholders there might be less than six months (or four months if the year is based on three four-monthly rotations) left to undertake other experience in the surgical specialties, psychiatry, anaesthetics and the like.

Another forceful part of the rhetoric surrounding the Foundation year has been the idea that trainees will have the opportunity to undertake 'taster periods' in specialties that they do not usually encounter in the early years of training, the objective being to support career planning. However, the sort of specialties where this might occur (radiology, pathology and anaesthetics, for example) would have to have F2 trainees on a supernumerary basis, as they would not be in a position to deliver service activity. It may be that some of the funding mentioned above will be available to support this, because it seems unlikely that this sort of activity could take place without funding to support it, any more than additional appointments for trainees in general practice can be made without funding.

## What to look for

We must all hope that the appointment process to the F2 year becomes resolved over the next year. Assuming this happens, it will not be too long before those people entering the F1 year as it rolls into action in August 2005 will be making their applications for an F2 year. It does seem that there are a few things that we can say about the rotations that will be available.

For many people, the idea of an opportunity to experience general practice is very attractive. Given that funding has been made available for this, it seems quite likely that F2 programmes including general practice may be quite widespread. This is one element that could be put into the process of choosing a rotation.

Some hospitals have been running pilot F2 rotations. The complex processes of assessment and appraisal that the F2 year demands may be better embedded in these hospitals than in others which are doing the programme for the first time. There will also be graduates of the pilot Foundation years available to ask about their experience.

If your driving ambition is to be a surgeon it obviously makes sense to apply for rotations which have a higher than average surgical content. It is clear that the new F2 programmes will have to be made up from previously existing SHO jobs. The service element of these posts will have to continue and it seems likely that some of them at least will be changed to F2 posts. The same consideration clearly applies for rotations including significant medicine or paediatrics content for those who are interested in these specialties. *The Next Steps*[1] suggests that experience in a particular specialty during the Foundation programme will not be a necessary precondition for entry into the early training programme for that specialty. This is a reasonable hope to express but in my view at least, potential candidates would be well advised to try and organize appropriate experience if they can.

Those specialties in which an inexperienced F2 trainee cannot offer any significant service delivery may or may not be able to offer a significant number of taster periods – it remains to be seen. This again might be an important element of the choice for some people.

Finally, it is probably sensible to try and make searching enquiries about any hospital you are interested in. The posts may be new but the general ethos of the hospital will not change much. If you know, for example, that both the previous A&E SHO posts and other posts such as the medical SHO posts were good in a particular hospital then it is likely that that hospital will be able to mount a reasonable F2 year.

---

### Box 3.3    What to look for in the F2 year

- A hospital where the generality of trainees feel well looked after and supported.
- A rotation that contains at least some of the specialties which you might be interested in; this may be easy for specialties such as A&E, medicine and general practice but more difficult for surgery, paediatrics and O&G.
- In some specialties (anaesthetics, pathology, psychiatry, radiology) you may have to search quite hard for 'taster experiences'.
- And finally, it may be a question of geography.

# And beyond?

If it is difficult to imagine what applying for an F2 year might be like, it is virtually impossible to see any further into the future. *The Next Steps* suggests that entry to specialist training will be competitive and that the grade will be a 'run-through grade' and that further competition will not be necessary following acceptance into the training programme. However, the document also acknowledges that 'a significant time period may be required' before the move to a new system is complete.

It is therefore very difficult to say what the landscape will look like as the first wave of trainees emerge from their Foundation programme. It is most likely that for the first few years at least, the system will look much as it does today, with trainees moving from the second Foundation year either into GP vocational schemes or into 'senior' SHO posts with a view to specialty training.

The best advice we can offer is to keep your eye on the plans as they develop. Relevant sources of information are shown in Box 3.4.

---

**Box 3.4    Sources of information**

- The Clinical Tutor and Postgraduate Centre staff in your hospital. Clinical Tutors have a network which gives them a good overview of events and rather more background than may be available in published material
- Website of the Royal College relevant to your probable career choice
- Local deanery website
- BMJ and BMA websites
- Postgraduate Medical Education and Training Board website: *www.pmetb.org.uk*
- Hospital doctor

---

The factors to be considered in selection of a post include:

- reputation of the organization, often acquired on the grapevine or by established repute and excellence
- contact with past or present post-holders leading to personal recommendations
- information included in the job description
- information on the hospital website: enlightened organizations are increasingly providing a good description of what is on offer on the Internet
- rotas including on-call commitments, cross-cover

- teaching and training provisions
- study leave
- facilities on site; library facilities out of hours
- track record of previous trainees
- type of clinical work undertaken
- research opportunities
- number of trainees
- accommodation
- family preferences

# References

1. Department of Health, Social Services and Public Safety, Scottish Executive, Welsh Assembly Government. *Modernizing Medical Careers – The Next Steps. The Future Shape of Foundation, Specialist and General Practice Training Programmes.* London: Department of Health, 2003.

# 4

# A career in primary care – all you wanted to know about general practice but were afraid to ask!

**Girish Malde**

This chapter will address the following areas.

- What is primary care?
- Definition of a GP
- Training requirements to be a GP
- Applying for general practice training
- Employment options in general practice
- How do GPs earn?
- Resources in primary care
- Opportunities in general practice

## What is primary care?

The provision of primary care has undergone a huge evolution since the NHS started in 1948. From the traditional single-handed and managed model, we are now moving to a managed primary care with doctors working in big practices alongside other practitioners, providing the care needed by the population they are serving. It will no longer be the traditional model of a doctor doing a surgery in the morning, having a leisurely lunch and afternoon nap followed by an evening surgery. Doctors are now working as a part of a multidisciplinary team providing fully comprehensive general medical services and managing chronic illnesses as well as disease prevention and health promotion.[1]

The Institute of Medicine's Primary Care Committee has produced an authoritative definition of primary care:

> 'Primary care is the provision of integrated, accessible healthcare services by clinicians who are accountable for addressing a large majority of personal healthcare needs, developing a sustained partnership with patients, and practising in the context of family and community.'

Hence primary care is a function. Healthcare professionals using knowledge and skills from various sources can contribute to achieving this function and often the best primary care is delivered by teams composed of individuals with a spectrum of expertise sufficient to respond to the needs and demands of their specific community. These teams may include nurses, physicians, administrators, receptionists, information assistants, social workers, physician assistants, mental health specialists and others with expertise relevant to the challenges faced by the people served by the primary care enterprise.

Primary care is the first port of call for 95% of people accessing healthcare in Britain. With the registered list system, primary care also has a gatekeeping role to other health services.

In the UK primary care is currently provided by teams led by general practitioners (GPs), in the majority of practices. Hence, at this time in the evolution of the NHS, GPs play a pivotal role in the provision of primary care.

## Definition of a GP

Many organizations, including the World Health Organization, have attempted to define what a GP is. The most appropriate definition is the one suggested by Olesen et al in their 2000 paper:[2]

> 'The general practitioner is a specialist trained to work in the front line of a healthcare system and to take the initial steps to provide care for any health problem(s) that patients may have. The general practitioner takes care of individuals in a society, irrespective of the patient's type of disease or other personal and social characteristics, and organizes the resources available in the healthcare system to the best advantage of the patients. The general practitioner engages with autonomous individuals across the fields of prevention, diagnosis, cure, care and palliation, using and integrating the sciences of biomedicine, medical psychology and medical sociology.'

# What are the requirements to be a GP?

---

### Box 4.1 Requirements to be a GP in the UK

- Full registration with the General Medical Council
- On the 'performer's list' of the relevant primary care trust
- Should hold JCPGTGP Certificate of Prescribed or Equivalent Experience

---

To work as a GP, you need full registration with the General Medical Council of the UK. Further details are available on the GMC website: *www.gmc-uk.org.uk*

All doctors working in general practice need to be on the 'performer's list' of their local primary care trust. It is important to apply to the PCT well in advance for this. This also applies to all doctors in training in general practice.

The GP needs to hold a Certificate of Prescribed or Equivalent Experience issued by the Joint Committee on Postgraduate Training in General Practice (JCPGTGP). The JCPGTGP oversees the education system for GPs in the UK and also issues certificates to newly qualified GPs. Further information is available on its website: *www.jcpgtgp.org.uk*. Its statutory functions are now being transferred to the Postgraduate Medical Education and Training Board (PMETB). There are no radical changes planned for the board in relation to GP training.

# Training requirements

---

### Box 4.2 Training requirements for primary care

- Three years after full or limited registration
- Up to 24 months in a recognized hospital job as an SHO
- Twelve months as a GP Registrar in a training practice
- Pass the Summative Assessment during the Registrar year

---

The minimum training requirement for general practice is three years after registration. The way things are at present, you need 24 months in approved hospital posts as a Senior House Officer and 12 months as a Registrar in general practice.

You can either do this by joining one of the three-year rotations offered by many local vocational training schemes or by organizing your own scheme.

This requires you to apply to an approved post in various specialties every six months. These posts should have both the College and the Postgraduate Dean's approval. The JCPGTGP prescribes the core specialties required as follows:

- general medicine
- care of elderly
- accident and emergency medicine or accident and emergency medicine with either general surgery or orthopaedic surgery
- obstetrics or gynaecology or obstetrics and gynaecology
- paediatrics
- psychiatry.

## GP Registrar

This is normally 12 months in an approved training practice under the supervision of a trainer. Appointment to a GP Registrar post may be part of the three-year vocational training scheme rotation or appointed directly by the deanery if you have done the training flexibly in a self-constructed scheme.

# How to apply for general practice training

After FY2, you can apply for a full three-year vocational training scheme. Each deanery will have details of each of the schemes on their websites.

All appointments to general practice training are now handled by the deaneries. There are 17 deaneries in the UK. There are two recruitment rounds each year for intakes in February and August. Further details on how to apply and the details of the vacancies and the schemes are available from the National Recruitment Office for General Practice Training website: *www.gprecruitment.org.uk*

## Application form

Doctors applying for a GP vocational scheme must first confirm that they are eligible for the post. In addition to the National Recruitment Office, all deaneries have their own websites and most of them provide a downloadable application pack. The above website has links to all the deaneries and through this to details of all the vocational schemes in each deanery.

It is important that you read the details of the application process, as the process is rigorous. The application and the interview process aim to be fair and choose the candidates who possess the competencies required to be a GP. Some deaneries have multiple choice and short answer questions as part of their filtering process.

All deaneries provide the opportunity to train flexibly or part time. For the hospital component of the training, you will need to secure funding from the deanery before you are appointed. Training in general practice as a flexible or part-time Registrar is not that problematic.

## Qualifying

The end point of training is the successful completion of the summative assessment, a national assessment taken during the GP Registrar year. There are four components:

- video assessment
- audit project
- MCQ paper
- trainer's structured report.

More information on the summative assessment can be found at: *www.nosa.org.uk*

Successful completion of the summative assessment and a Certificate of Prescribed or Equivalent Experience show that the doctor has reached a satisfactory level of competence and may practise as a GP.

At present the MRCGP examination is optional and most Registrars do it at the end of their Registrar year or within 2–3 years of this. It is not a requirement to sit the MRCGP examination as an exit examination.

# Employment options in general practice

Broadly speaking, there are two ways you can be employed in general practice. One is the traditional self-employed independent contractor and the second is being employed as a salaried general practitioner.

## Self-employed independent contractor: GP principal

The traditional pathway once you have completed the training has been to become a full-time, self-employed general practitioner principal. You would buy into a traditional partnership or take up a practice as a single-handed practitioner. In either case you would be providing all the necessary medical care to your patients as well as running a small business. This would involve some management-related work in the practice. You would be responsible for employment of all your staff as well as owning the premises and a share in the business. With the new GP Contract, self-employment is becoming rarer, as more and more practices are looking to employ doctors as salaried GPs.

## Salaried general practitioners

The demographics of the workforce are changing and many young doctors are choosing to work in a salaried position that gives them a lot of flexibility. It allows them to work part time and take up other types of jobs that a general practice career can offer.

Qualified GPs can be employed directly by practices or by PCTs or other organizations providing primary care. The advantage of being salaried is that you are an employee and hence may not have the same responsibilities as the principal. There is no national payscale for salaried GPs at present, though the BMA has issued a guidance salary scale. The salary has to be negotiated with the employer organization.

You have the options of being employed full time, part time or flexibly and can balance work and life very well. This option is more attractive to many doctors with a young and growing family.

# How do general practitioners earn?

In terms of contract status, there are two types of practice that you will come across. One is the General Medical Services (GMS) practice and the other is the Personal Medical Services (PMS) practice.

## GMS practice

These practices work under the contract set nationally and negotiated by the General Practitioner Committee of the BMA. The new GMS Contract was implemented on 1 April 2004. Before this, income was based on the 'red book', a manual of fees and allowances, and the income of the practice was based on its list size as well as on claiming fees for providing extra services such as contraception, maternity care, vaccinations and immunizations, cervical cytology, night visits, temporary residents, etc. It was up to the practice to ensure that all possible claimable services were provided and claimed for. With the new GMS Contract, practices no longer have to do this as the payment in now included in the global sum.

## PMS practice

Prior to the new contract, practices could agree a contract with their primary care organization. This gave practices room to work in an innovative way to provide services that their population needed. To help practices to achieve this, they were given growth money to employ salaried general practitioners or nurse practitioners.

The PMS practices had all their item-of-service payments included in the gross contract and hence were no longer required to claim individually for the services provided. This certainly reduced the paperwork that most doctors were complaining about.

At present, both the GMS and PMS practices are paid in a very similar way, based on the practice's historical earnings and other formulae.

Broadly speaking, the way practices are paid is as follows.

- Global sum
- Additional services
- Enhanced services
  - National enhanced services
  - Direct enhanced services
  - Local enhanced services
- Providing quality services (quality and outcomes payment)
- Other

## Global sum

This is paid for providing essential medical services and additional services. The essential medical services include:

- management of patients who are ill or think they are ill
- management of terminal illness
- chronic disease management.

The global sum includes the payments that were part of the old GMS Contract being paid as per the 'red book':

- basic practice allowance
- capitation fees
- night allowance and visit fees
- health promotion payments (excluding chronic disease management)
- temporary residents
- deprivation payments
- registration fees

- postgraduate education allowance
- practice staff reimbursements.

The global sum is calculated on the Carr-Hill formula and is based on the following indices for each practice:

- age/sex indices
- nursing and residential patient factor
- morbidity and mortality
- new patient weighting
- additional needs weighting (postcode)
- unavoidable costs (staff) practice postcodes.

## Additional services

The global sum also includes payments for additional services as below:

- cervical screening
- contraceptive services
- vaccinations and immunizations
- child health surveillance
- maternity services
- minor surgery (part)
- childhood vaccinations and immunizations.

If the practice opts out of providing the above additional services, the global sum is reduced accordingly.

## Enhanced services

These are defined as either the essential or additional services as above but provided to a much higher standard (e.g. extended minor surgery) or services that do not form part of essential or additional services. These services are commissioned and paid for by the primary care organization and include the following.

- National enhanced services
  - Alcohol misuse
  - Anticoagulation monitoring
  - IUCD fitting
  - Patients with depression
  - Immediate care/first response care

- Care of the homeless
- Intrapartum care
- Minor injury services
- Sexual health services
- Multiple sclerosis patients
- Near patient testing
- Direct enhanced services
  - Improved access scheme
  - Childhood immunizations
  - Influenza and pneumococcal vaccination
  - Quality information preparation
  - Dealing with violent patients
  - Minor surgery
- Local enhanced services
  - Minor injuries
  - Dressings, suture removals, hospital scripts
  - Anticoagulation monitoring and near patient testing
  - Minor surgery (maximum 25 procedures per principal per year; includes incisions, injections and HRT implants etc.)
  - Zoladex administration
  - Substance misuse

## Rewarding practices for quality and outcome

The new contract has allowed practices to provide quality services, both clinical and organizational, to their patients. On achieving the target levels of these services, practices are rewarded by extra payments based on points achieved. A practice can achieve a maximum of 1050 points, based on the following.

- Clinical indicators           550
- Organizational indicators     184
- Additional services            36
- Patient experience            100
- Holistic care payments        100
- Quality practice payments      30
- Access bonus                   50
- **Total**                    **1050**

In the first year of the new contract, practices were paid £75.00 for each point achieved based on an average practice size of 5891 patients. Larger practices would earn more proportionally compared to small practices.

## *Other income*

Apart from their main income, many practices can boost their earnings by doing other work.

- Training grants for training GP Registrars
- Medical student teaching
- Training other doctors
- Doing medical reports such as:
  - Insurance reports
  - DSS reports
  - Solicitors' reports
  - Occupational
- Completing forms such as:
  - passports/driving licence applications
  - health insurance verification forms

The rates of pay for these extra services are determined annually and can be found on the BMA website or in *Medeconomics*, which is a monthly GP magazine.

# Resources in primary care

As defined above, primary care is a function and is best provided in teams to meet the needs of the population it serves. The primary care team may comprise:

- GPs
- practice nurses and nurse practitioners
- counsellors/psychologists
- chiropodists
- dietitians
- physiotherapists
- acupuncturists
- osteopaths
- midwives
- health visitors
- district nurses
- community psychiatric nurses
- Macmillan nurses
- specialist nurses.

An effective team relies on each of the above providing the necessary services and hence dealing with most problems in the community.

# Opportunities in general practice

General practice can be a very good portfolio career as there is a lot of flexibility and you can choose how you want to work, when you want to work and what else you want to do apart from providing general medical services. Some of the many opportunities available to GPs are listed below.[3]

## *General practitioners with special interest: GPSi*

With more and more care being provided in primary care and with an emphasis on developing intermediate care, more and more GPs are developing their special skills to work as GPSi. These are posts created within PCTs to meet the needs of the *local* population and provide easily accessible care at an intermediate level. It is hoped that they will help to reduce referrals to hospitals and hence reduce waiting times all round.

GPSi normally work in the community, taking direct referrals from GP colleagues. There are GPSi posts in various specialties including musculoskeletal medicine, dermatology, diabetes, ENT, genitourinary and sexual health, etc.

## *Clinical assistant posts*

GPs who wish to develop a specialist interest in a hospital specialty can work as clinical assistants, employed by the hospital and paid on a sessional rate. Clinical assistant posts exist in many specialties including A&E, diabetes, endocrinology, ENT, dermatology, palliative care, etc. Your local hospital is the best place to approach for such opportunities.

## *Primary care trust work*

### Management

GP advisors on the Professional Executive Committee of the PCT Management Board or as medical leads in the locality. Medical Directors in most PCTs are general practitioners. They are responsible for the clinical governance issues in general practice.

### Appraisers

With the need for annual GP appraisal, there is plenty of opportunity for GPs to train as appraisers and work for the PCT.

Quality and Outcome Framework assessors

With the new contract and the practices needing to achieve quality points to generate income, the PCT's assessing team need GPs as leaders.

Employed as GPs by PCT

Many PCTs need to employ GPs directly to boost the local workforce as well as help with struggling practices.

## Out-of-hours GPs

Since GPs are now able to opt out of providing out-of-hours care, many out-of-hours organizations need to employ GPs to do sessional work. Many GPs take this option in the early stages of their career, to boost their income as well as enjoying the variety of clinical care experiences it provides.

## Complementary medicine

General practitioners can train to provide complementary therapies such as acupuncture, homeopathy and hypnotherapy, etc. These services can be provided on the NHS, providing the primary care organization agrees to fund them, or they can be offered on a private basis. Many GPs enjoy practising these alternative therapies.

## Forensic medicine

- *Forensic physicians*: also known as police surgeons or forensic medical examiners, these are mostly GPs with a part-time contract with the police force.
- *Prison doctors*: these are GPs employed by the Home Office, providing medical services in prisons.

## Sports and exercise medicine

Doctors can work in sports injury clinics, as a professional club doctor or as full-time professional athletics physicians. Most posts are part time and are usually undertaken by GPs. Further qualifications can be achieved and details are mentioned in Chambers *et al.*[3]

## Occupational health

After gaining extra qualifications, many GPs provide occupational health services to local organizations. This is usually done on a sessional basis.

## Education

There are plenty of opportunities available for providing education in primary care.

### Medical student teaching

The current medical school curriculum includes teaching and placements based in primary care and local medical schools are always looking for practices and GPs to provide this education.

### GP Registrar trainer

GP Registrars are required to do at least 12 months of their training with an approved trainer based in an approved training practice. Approval for the practice and the trainer is normally granted by the local deanery. There are minimum standards required of the practice and the trainer and all the details are available on the local deanery website.

### Vocational training scheme course organizers

Again appointed by the local deanery to provide training for future GPs.

### General practice tutors

These posts are appointed by the deanery to plan and organize continuing postgraduate education for GPs in each area.

## Academic medicine and research

Though research in general practice is not as widespread as in hospital medicine, more and more research opportunities are now available in primary care. GPs interested in doing this can do research in their own time or join a local network that will provide training and funding to conduct GP research.

There are some opportunities available in the Department of General Practice of medical schools. These departments may have an attached general practice. If you are interested in academia, you can apply for employment in such practices with opportunities to do research.

## Writing and media work

General practitioners do a lot of television and radio work, giving medical input to various health-related issues and programmes. Writing for popular papers and weekly magazines is also an important opportunity.

# Conclusion

General practice offers a varied and challenging opportunity as a career. The normal course is a three-year specialist training in an approved scheme after the second Foundation year. Though the MRCGP is not an essential exit examination for all GPs in training, more and more trainees are taking it during their training year or immediately after. There are different career pathways available to GPs and you can choose the option most appropriate to you. General practice offers flexible working and there is plenty of opportunity to supplement income by providing extra services in the practice. Apart from providing traditional general medical care, GPs have many other options to make their career varied and exciting.

# References

1. Jones R, Britten N, Culpepper L *et* al. *Oxford Textbook of Primary Medical Care*. Oxford: Oxford University Press, 2003.
2. Olesen F, Dickinson J, Hjortdahl P. General practice – a time for a new definition. *Br Med J* 2000; **320:** 354–7.
3. Chambers R, Mohanna K, Field SJ. *Opportunities and Options in Medical Careers*. Oxford: Radcliffe Medical Press, 2000.

# Useful websites

*www.gprecruitment.org.uk* National Recruitment Office for General Practice Training

*www.jcpgtgp.org.uk* Joint Committee for Postgraduate Training in General Practice

*www.gmc-uk.org.uk* General Medical Council

*www.rcgp.org.uk* Royal College of General Practitioners

*www.bma.org.uk* British Medical Association

*www.nosa.org.uk* National Office for Summative Assessment

## Definition

The commonest definition of clinical governance is the following:

'A framework through which NHS organizations are accountable for continually improving the quality of their services and safeguarding high standards of care by creating an environment in which excellence in clinical care will flourish.'[1]

In simpler language, this means the structures employed by trusts and clinicians to deliver a constantly improving high degree of care for which they are responsible.

## The seven pillars of clinical governance

- *Staff management*: trusts have a duty to ensure that the staff employed are sufficiently trained and accredited in their area of expertise and that their practices comply with current standards in their profession.
- *Education and training*: it is incumbent upon staff to ensure they have the appropriate competencies to perform the job for which they are employed and that these are continually updated.
- *Patient and public involvement*: patients' input in organizing the services they access should be actively encouraged and their views solicited on how services should develop.
- *Complaints and clinical risk*: problem identification and a proactive process of interdiction should be the norm. And if problems do arise, learning from the experience is desirable.
- *Clinical audit*: this serves to maintain a minimum high standard of practice as compared to a benchmark.

- *Research and effectiveness*: evidence-based practice is a key element of this approach to develop and test new ideas and techniques and to integrate them into current practice if they prove advantageous.
- *Information management and technology*: a comparative performance check against what happened in the past and what exists in other organizations is facilitated through the appropriate and effective employment of these tools.

A useful acronym to recall these factors is **PRRICES**:

**P**atient involvement
**R**isk management
**R**esearch and education
**I**nformation management
**C**linical audit
**E**ducation, training and development
**S**taff involvement

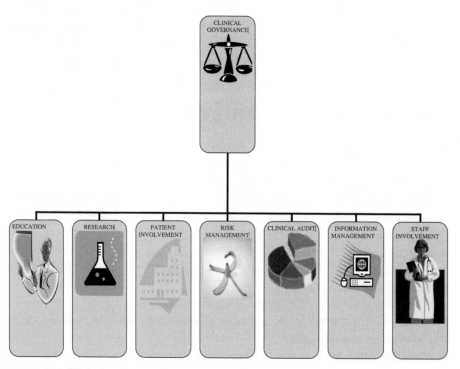

FIGURE 5.1    Clinical governance

# Introduction

In the United Kingdom clinical governance was introduced in 1998 as a systematic approach to the delivery of high-quality healthcare. A duty of quality was placed on NHS organizations in the 1999 NHS Act. This introduced corporate accountability for clinical quality and performance. Clinical governance is a 'system-wide' process which has a number of features, to be explored further in this chapter.

Though it appears that clinical governance is a new invention, its essence has been around since time immemorial. Every advance in medical practice, from the first blood transfusion in 1829 to the pioneering use of chloroform as an anaesthetic by James Simpson in 1847, to the 1928 announcement of the discovery of penicillin by Alexander Fleming and subsequent introduction of anti-polio vaccination in 1956, has been part of the drive to improve the way in which we practise our craft. Each has encompassed some of the elements of clinical governance in the move to explore and exploit new technologies of their time.

More modern developments, such as the first heart transplant in Cape Town in 1967, the birth in 1978 of the world's first test tube baby, Louise Joy Brown, the discovery of HIV in 1984 and the success of the Human Genome Project in deciphering the 3.1 billion subunits of human DNA in 2000, will for decades to come challenge our knowledge and skills in medicine. They will better serve all of humanity by applying the structures of clinical governance in finessing the positive aspects of these revolutionary achievements.

These represent but a sample of the progress that our scientific field has made. However, a lack of structure has impaired the benefits derived from these pioneering discoveries.

Under the aegis of clinical governance:

- the best evidence is gathered and applied
- there is meaningful contribution from patients so that the therapies derived are tailored to need
- there is rigorous training in application of treatments
- there are systems of feedback and supervision to minimize risk
- there is a system of information technology and data storage and transfer, enabling efficiency.

Thus we should expect more scientifically rigorous and expeditious gain benefiting those whom we serve.

By encouraging a structured approach in which the successes of others can be communicated to all, we can accelerate the modernization of healthcare.

This is where clinical governance permits, promotes and promulgates perfection in the profession.

## Participants in clinical governance

Apart from our individual responsibilities as physicians, which will be underscored later, there is a plethora of organizations tasked with the responsibility of ensuring good clinical governance across the NHS. The very seminal step in the process of creating the staff and particularly the doctors by whom the NHS will function cohesively and competently has become subsumed in the drive to modernization.

The major players include:

- local NHS trust
- National Institute for Clinical Excellence (NICE)
- National Service Frameworks (NSFs)
- Commission for Health Improvement (CHI) (Healthcare Commission)
- Clinical Governance Support Team (CGST)
- NHS Modernization Agency
- the various Royal Colleges
- Department of Health (DoH)
- General Medical Council (GMC)
- British Medical Association (BMA)
- Patient Advocacy and Liaison Service (PALS)
- Higher Education Funding Council Committee.

### At trust level

Within each trust the Chief Executive is ultimately responsible. This is an extension of corporate responsibility and ensures that not only are financial and service considerations represented but additionally, the quality of care provided is of a high standard and a criterion of equal importance.

Senior clinicians are expected to ensure that on a daily basis, good clinical practice is pursued and should identify any problems in the system and address them in a meaningful fashion. Should these challenges prove beyond the capabilities of the clinician, then they should inform those within the organization who are better equipped to offer solutions.

Each physician should actively participate in this process of quality assurance. Where a persistent problem is identified, efforts should be made to rectify it in conjunction with the management team within whose remit it normally falls.

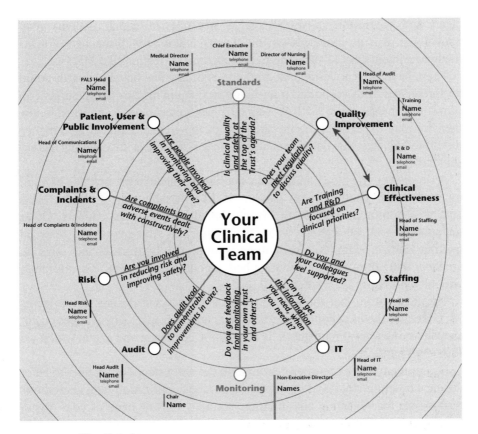

**FIGURE 5.2** The clinical team

We must all take ownership of the entire structure within which we train and through which we execute our professional responsibilities. It is no longer acceptable to excuse ourselves from its failings if we are in a position to effect change.

As a physician in the modern NHS, each individual should endeavour to be as professional as possible, to practise safely, to a high standard, and to be able to work effectively in a health organization committed to clinical governance.

Health organizations are to become truly patient centred by considering and providing for diversity of culture, ethnicity, race, religion and sexuality. They should also establish clear systems and methods for assuring and improving quality and by promoting teamwork and high standards of practice. Additionally a key element in the quality of healthcare is patient safety.

With the emergence of the 'superbug' MRSA (methicillin-resistant *Staphylococcus aureus*), trusts have awakened to the absolute need to create a clean and environmentally risk-averse structure in which patients may convalesce. It is no longer defensible that a patient be well managed for his medical ailment only to succumb to a nosocomial infection like MRSA.

There have been governmental mutterings of late that hospital boards could be threatened with corporate manslaughter charges if they are negligent in preventing the spread of MRSA. If such a proposal becomes established in law then we may expect it to be the thin end of the wedge. Clinical governance therefore dictates the definitive allocation of resources to ensuring safety standards.

A simple yet effective contribution we may all make in the practice of good hygiene in our dealings with patients is hand washing on a regular basis and, at a minimum, the use of alcohol-based gels between patients. Other undemanding efforts include wearing tie clips/pins (this avoids the material making contact with one patient and subsequently transferring bugs to another), not sitting on the patient's bed, cleaning equipment, e.g. slit lamp, with alcohol wipes after use, and so on.

The recognition that the solution is to establish and design safe systems which reduce the likelihood of medical error and its impact when it does occur, as well as to learn from mistakes, is a welcome challenge and one in which we should all participate.

Equipping today's health professional in the early stages of training to enter this new environment should be a priority for the organizations and institutions responsible for education and training. You may thus demand of your trust a minimum in terms of equipment, facilities and resources so that your training and service commitments coexist complementarily.

Where these demands are reasonable and unresolved after negotiation, there should be recourse to a lobbying group such as the BMA or the deanery where a training post is being pursued. Trusts have a tendency to listen to these bodies, especially where their training accreditation may be revoked.

## What's your role as the physician?

Clinical governance should enable you to meet the challenge of the changing health and healthcare needs of our increasingly ageing, fattening and medically dependent population. You should not consider it an onerous impediment in your professional undertakings but embrace its ethos in a new way of working that is now affecting the NHS.

In what may have appeared as an alien concept to our predecessors and even those who entered the profession just two decades ago, the individual clinician is accountable through the corporate management structure and bound (albeit informally) to meet the goals and contractual commitments of the trust in whose employ she or he practises.

The modern physician participates in a team increasingly led by a clinical manager and shares accountability for meeting the team's service delivery goals. She or he should perform diligently the tasks for which remuneration is gained.

Patients are becoming ever more aware and demanding and this should encourage us to develop communication skills which permit us to listen, understand and empathize but particularly pre-empt common sources of complaint. You may readily pick up on cues once you have learned to be attuned to them.

Informed consent has become a cornerstone of the doctor–patient interaction whenever we wish to intrude upon the person physically. We should take sufficient time to inform the patient about exactly or approximately what will transpire and possible delays, shortcomings, risks, adverse effects and, at the extreme, the possibility of death.

Where a consultation is troubled, every effort should be employed to regain harmony. It may be by taking time out, offering an excuse such as the need to attend to a more pressing case or to retrieve some further information like blood results. During this respite, discuss the matter with colleagues or seniors who may be able to offer an alternative approach or intervene to alleviate the situation.

If a situation becomes threatening then raise an alarm and exit as quickly as possible. Never become physically involved in an affray as it may ensnare you in subsequent criminal proceedings.

Even a consultant needs assistance on occasion even if she or he may be loath to admit it. Therefore it is expected that if you find yourself in a situation where your skills and knowledge are insufficient to address the task in hand, you should solicit the input of a senior. There is no heroism in inadequacy.

Rigorous documentation is also essential. Remember, if it is not written down, it didn't happen. There are protocols in place in many trusts regarding the salient information to be gathered, depending on the case type. It is your obligation to familiarize yourself with these.

It may seem self-evident but remember to maintain good hygiene and be appropriately attired when dealing with patients. You are an ambassador for your trust and profession and when a patient is disgruntled, he or she may generalize to all of the staff as having or lacking the attributes that triggered complaint.

As a professional in the science of medicine, your contribution is invaluable in the daily functioning of your trust. If you must be absent for unforeseen circumstances, it is incumbent upon you to give as much notice to your employer as possible so that a substitute practitioner may be sought. Also you should attempt to minimize any adverse impact to the routine of your performance by managing your social engagements in an appropriate manner.

It is not acceptable to turn up for work inebriated or with any perceptible after-effects of over-indulgence in ethanol. A minimum of eight hours is recommended between cessation of drinking and commencement of a shift, especially where you will exceed the prescribed quantity permissible to drive.

Considerable outlay and sometimes sacrifice are involved in the provision of scheduled training, not counting that doctors in training are generally paid as part of their contract. We should thus be responsible in attending these sessions and prepare beforehand so as to maximize the learning experience.

Participation in audit is now mandatory for all doctors in training and this may serve as a springboard to pursue interests in research. It is an outdated notion that you have to be academically inclined to be involved in research. There are many simple projects around to which you may contribute.

In the final analysis, you should be able to practise your skill to a very high standard, through being able to appraise and use evidence (by critical appraisal of journal papers and information searches on databases like Cochrane and Medline), becoming a life-long learner (continuing medical education), maintaining professional standards (this will be assessed through regular appraisal) and being an effective team member and leader.

We need to understand the value of partnership and communication with patients, colleagues and members of allied professional groups. A commitment to and skill in promoting health, preventing illness, diagnosing and treating injury and disease, and caring for people with chronic sickness and disability should be fostered in the new structures of working.

Key messages

- Have a sense of corporate responsibility
- Communicate effectively
- Ensure consent is informed, including adequate risk appraisal
- Avoid confrontation
- Know your limitations and seek advice when out of your depth
- Make sure you document all necessary and relevant matters
- Be professional at all times
- Endeavour to be a team player
- Constantly improve and refine your clinical knowledge and skills
- Participate in audits and research at every available opportunity

## *Some other players in clinical governance*

National Institute for Clinical Excellence

This institution established in 1999 works on behalf of the NHS and the people who use it. It makes recommendations on treatments and care using the best available evidence.

Currently the NICE produces guidance in three areas of health.

- *Technology appraisals*: guidance on the use of new and existing medicines and treatments within the NHS in England and Wales.
- *Clinical guidelines*: guidance on the appropriate treatment and care of people with specific diseases and conditions within the NHS in England and Wales.
- *Interventional procedures*: guidance on whether interventional procedures used for diagnosis or treatment are safe enough and work well enough for routine use in England, Wales and Scotland.

Published guidelines include:

- chronic heart failure, second programme July 2003 to July 2007
- chronic obstructive pulmonary disease, sixth wave February 2004 to February 2008
- head injury, second programme June 2003 to June 2007
- type 1 diabetes, second programme July 2004 to July 2008.


National Service Frameworks

NSFs are long-term strategies elaborated by the Department of Health for improving specific areas of care. They establish measurable goals within set time frames and promulgate ways to ensure their progress. They serve to raise quality and decrease variations in service. Launched in April 1998, they cover the following.

- *Coronary heart disease*: this NSF launched in March 2000 sets 12 standards to be implemented over a 10-year period, for improved prevention, diagnosis and treatment, and goals to secure fair access to high-quality services.
- *Cancer*: the NHS Cancer Plan (September 2000) provides the fullest statement of the government's comprehensive national programme for investment and reform of cancer services in England.
- *Paediatric intensive care*: the NSF for paediatric intensive care was established in 1999.
- *Mental health*: another NSF launched in 1999, which describes how mental health services will be planned, delivered and monitored until 2009 and lists

seven standards that set targets for the mental healthcare of adults aged up to 65 years. These standards concern health promotion and stigma, primary care and access to specialist services, needs of those with severe and enduring mental illness, carers' needs and suicide reduction.

- *Older people*: the NSF for older people was published in March 2001. It sets new national standards and service models of care across health and social services for all senior citizens whether they live at home or in residential care or are being cared for in hospital.
- *Diabetes*: currently 1.3 million people in England suffer from diabetes and the number is rising. The diabetes NSF is a concerted effort to ensure a homogenous and excellent standard of care despite a patient's postcode.
- *Long-term conditions*: the NSF for long-term conditions, published in March 2005, aims to improve the lives of the many people who live with neurological and other chronic conditions by providing them with better health and social care services.

Other NSFs concern renal services, paediatric care and the involvement of the pharmaceutical industry.

## Healthcare Commission

Formerly referred to as the Commission for Healthcare Improvement (CHI), the Healthcare Commission promotes improvement in the quality of the NHS and independent healthcare. Its responsibilities are all aimed at improving the quality of healthcare. It has a statutory duty to assess the performance of healthcare organizations, award annual performance ratings for the NHS and co-ordinate reviews of healthcare by other bodies.

## General Medical Council

The GMC was established under the Medical Act of 1858. Its stated vision is 'to be recognized as delivering and safeguarding the highest standards of medical ethics, education and practice, in the interests of patients, public and the profession'. It exists not to protect the medical profession but to defend the interests of patients.

## Patient Advice and Liaison Service

PALS offers confidential help, advice and support to patients, relatives and carers, and helps to guide them through the different services available from the NHS. It focuses on improving the service to NHS patients by helping to sort out problems and answer questions about local health services. PALS does not replace the existing complaints procedure

In most NHS trusts its remit is to:

- advise and support patients, their families and carers.
- furnish information on NHS services
- listen to the concerns, suggestions or queries and feedback comments and trends to trust committee service providers.
- assist in problem resolution in a timely manner on behalf of the patient.

NHS Modernization Agency

The NHS MA was established in April 2001 and is designed to support the NHS and its partner organizations in the task of modernizing services and improving experiences and outcomes for patients. It has focused on improving access, increasing local support, raising standards of care and capturing and sharing knowledge widely.

# The patient-centred approach

In today's NHS, patients have a realization of themselves as true consumers of a service which they, as taxpayers, fund. They expect to be respected, to be empowered with information to enable them to make informed choices, and to become equal partners in decisions about their case.

Following the debacles of the children's heart surgery service in Bristol and the uninformed removal of children's organs after autopsy at Alder Hey Hospital in Liverpool and other centres, the physician, if she or he was still foolishly self-deluded, has been disabused of any notion of God-like status.

Patient complaints should be dealt with in a timely fashion as stipulated by current complaint procedures and where it is warranted, an apology should be offered. If the complaint is only at the vocal stage, endeavours to resolve the situation before escalation to a more formal forum may be undertaken. However, at times it is necessary to allow a complaint to progress through the system as it may highlight specific concerns which it is in the clinician's interest to amplify.

NHS trusts must be clear about how information and feedback from patients past and present is used to assess and advance the quality of services. By empowering patients with relevant information and increasing their contribution to planning services, the progress of clinical governance can be accelerated. Their input will permit a responsive system that prioritizes according to their needs yet maintains a high level of quality.

# Conclusion

The delivery of modern healthcare in this century requires a new kind of health professional. This person needs to be outfitted, through her or his own preparations but also those facilitated by the organization, with the capabilities to surpass the conventional doctor–patient relationship and achieve a new level of partnership with patients.

Additionally, the ability to lead, manage and work effectively in a team and organizational environment, practise safe high-quality care but also constantly create the opportunities for improvement should be engendered.

We must in partnership establish a functional, cohesive and competent team of practitioners with capable and possibly visionary leaders at the helm. An NHS that functions as a healthy organization matters to patients.

The challenge of clinical governance is to transform the culture and service delivery of NHS organizations throughout the UK. It is a big, bold and beneficial initiative that has shown that it can inspire and enthuse. Given sufficient nurturing, it will transform the modern practice of medical science with barely imagined gains and have the surest support of patients whose input is integral. It will make us proud as physicians.

Embrace the transformation.

# Reference

1. Scally G, Donaldson LJ. Clinical governance and the drive for quality improvement in the new NHS in England. *Br Med J* 1998; 4 July: 61–5.

# Useful websites

Standards

*www.dh.gov.uk* National Service Frameworks
*www.nice.org.uk* National Institute for Clinical Excellence
*www.dh.gov.uk* Policy (Department of Health)
*www.nhsia.nhs.uk/phsmi/clinicalgovernance* Professional Bodies

Patient, user and public involvement

*www. cppih.org* Commission for Patient and Public Involvement in Health

*www.chi.nhs.uk* Commissions for Health Improvement
*www.chai.org.uk* Commission for Healthcare Audit and Inspection
*www.dh.gov.uk* Department of Health

Quality improvement

*www.cgsupport.nhs.uk* Clinical Governance Support Team
*www.modern.nhs.uk* Modernization Agency

Clinical effectiveness

*www.nhsu.nhs.uk* NHS University
*www.nelh.nhs.uk* National Electronic Library for Health
*www.nks.nhs.uk* National Knowledge Service
*www.dh.gov.uk* Department of Health Research Directorate

Complaints and incidents

*www.drfoster.co.uk* Dr Foster
*www.dh.gov.uk* NHS complaints figure and maternal deaths
*www.npsa.org.uk* National Patient Safety Agency
*www.ncepod.nhs.uk* Perioperative deaths
*www.cesdi.org.uk* Infant deaths

Risk

*www.dh.gov.uk* Controls assurance
*www.casu.org.uk* Controls Assurance Support Unit
*www.nhsla.co.uk* Clinical Negligence Scheme for Trusts
*www.nhs.uk/localnhsservices* Local Commissioners

Audit

*www.nhsia.nhs.uk/phsmi/pages/ncasp.asp* National Clinical Audit Support
Programme
*www.audit-commission.gov.uk* Audit Commission
*www.dh.gov.uk* Department of Health

Monitoring

*www.chi.nhs.uk* Commissions for Health Improvement

*www.dh.gov.uk* Social Services Inspectorate
*www.mhac.trent.nhs.uk* Mental Health Act Commission

## Staffing

*www.dh.gov.uk* Workforce Development Confederations
*www.ncaa.nhs.uk* National Clinical Assessment Authority
*www.gmc-uk.org* Professional Bodies/Registration
*www.nmc-uk.org* Professional Bodies/Registration

## Information technology

*www.dh.gov.uk* Central Statistical Returns Office and Information Policy Unit
*www.nhsia.nhs.uk* NHS Information Authority

# 6 Appraisal

## Gordon Jackson

Appraisal now forms part of the life of every doctor in the UK. For trained doctors in any career post, regular appraisal is part of the revalidation process which will in future be required of all doctors in order to practise. This sort of appraisal is concerned with ensuring that trained doctors – hospital consultants and non-consultant grade doctors, GPs, occupational health physicians and all other practising doctors – are maintaining good standards of medical practice.

For the trainee, appraisal must fulfil this purpose and must also provide a support to appropriate progression through a training programme. Strictly speaking, it may be more appropriate to talk about 'educational appraisal' for the activities involved in monitoring and supporting a trainee's progress through the Foundation years, with ordinary or employment appraisal being the element necessary for a doctor to validate their registration. In practice, the two processes will probably take place simultaneously.

An important part of training in the Foundation years is that trainees themselves will be responsible for ensuring that their appraisals take place and for ensuring that the documentation is completed.

## Appraisal, assessment and evaluation

In everyday English, these words might all be taken to mean much the same thing. However, in the world of education they have distinct meanings, and the distinction is useful.

- *Assessment*: exams and the like.
- *Appraisal*: a process involving feedback on performance and achievement of previously set goals.

- *Evaluation*: a process of enquiry designed to explore the effectiveness of a training course or a training event. Evaluation is therefore about the process and the institution in which it takes place, rather than about trainees themselves.

Success in all these activities depends upon those taking part understanding what they are engaged upon. Conversations can get both convoluted and confusing when one party thinks the discussion is an appraisal whilst the other thinks it is an evaluation of the post.

## Appraisal and assessment – what's the difference?

### Assessment

There are many published definitions of assessment. However, the key element of assessment is that it is a process designed to form a judgement about an individual's ability in a particular sphere of activity. The purpose of the judgement is to provide information to others about the individual's knowledge, skills and (if possible and necessary) attitudes in the particular sphere. Thus universities and employers are able to form judgements about skills and knowledge in mathematics from assessments such as maths GCSE and A level.

In a medical context, the fundamental purpose of all assessments is to provide an assurance that the individual has the knowledge, skills and attitudes appropriate to practise medicine in the arena in which they work. At base, the purpose of an assessment is always to provide an assurance for members of the public that their doctors are what they say they are, and do have the appropriate skills and knowledge to do what they are planning to do. Thus universities examine medical students under the aegis of the GMC in order for students to qualify for admission to the Medical Register.

In the Foundation years the plan is to use well-validated techniques such as $360°$ appraisal, directly observed procedures and structured case discussions to assess progress. The good news is that from the experience of pilot studies so far, it appears that both trainers and trainees find these assessments valuable as guides to further learning and development.

### Appraisal

Appraisal has a different aim from assessment. The fundamental purpose is to evaluate an individual's performance against an agreed set of objectives. So appraisal is there for individuals and for the organizations in which they work.

In industrial management, appraisals may be directed towards the achievement of targets and an individual's pay may be based on the outcome of appraisal. This sort of appraisal is therefore driven by the needs of the organization, with any benefits for the individual being subservient to this aim.

In contrast, for trainees in medicine, appraisal should usually be directed towards educational goals so that appraisal is there for the benefit of the trainee. Appraisal should be all about processes such as feedback on performance, planning future educational activity, planning future service activity and so on, all for the benefit of the trainee.

Thus it is clearly possible to pass or fail an assessment but the words 'pass' and 'fail' should have no meaning in the context of appraisal. Indeed, even the words 'good' and 'bad' have to be used very cautiously: a trainee who has not done very well over previous months may have a very good and successful appraisal if, on going through things with the appraiser, they are able to identify problems and, better still, find solutions for them. It is self-evident that the process would be quite tough for both parties and 'bad' in that sense; however, if the outcomes are good then it would have been one of the most successful of all appraisals. (It is really quite easy to give feedback to people who are doing well; it is much more testing to impart bad news and still have a positive effect.)

## Appraisal 'links to' assessment[1]

Though appraisal and assessment have different purposes, there are strong links between them. Feedback on assessments clearly has a significant role to play in an individual's progress through the grade. For those who are doing well, it is very helpful for them to know about it. For those who have problems, a more structured and formal system of assessment of performance will enable both trainees and their assessors to pinpoint areas of difficulty and to come up with a plan to improve things.

The reverse link is more problematic and as a general rule, the process of appraisal is best kept as a confidential discussion between the trainee and the appraiser and should not feed into the assessment process.

Newer forms of assessment such as directly observed procedures, case note review and case-based discussion will certainly be used in the Foundation years. These have been well validated in healthcare systems outside the UK and both trainees and trainers find them valuable. However, if the assessor is also an appraiser for the trainee concerned, there may be some difficulty in maintaining a clear distinction between the different sorts of conversation. At any one time, trainer and trainee might be:

- undertaking assessment: 'You did well, and you have certainly passed this assessment'
- concerned with feedback on performance in that particular assessment: '...things would have been easier for you if you had concentrated a bit more on the nature of the pain and had picked up that it was pleuritic'
- concerned with overall appraisal on performance: 'You remember that we had some concerns about your history taking before. Do you feel this is improving ... ?'

The matter will be more complicated still if evaluation is thrown in on top of appraisal and assessment:

- ' I think this case is a bit complex for someone at your stage. I wonder if we wouldn't have been better to do a straightforward MI'

The trick to success in this is for the trainer to be quite clear about which part of the process is going on at any particular time.

## Who is my appraiser?

There are no fixed rules about who is responsible for appraisal of foundation trainees. Individual postgraduate deaneries will probably be responsible for setting the rules within their own patch although this is not yet decided. However, there are a number of things which the appraisal process will have to deliver.

Feedback on clinical performance can only be given by someone who is part of the clinical team. However, the other objectives sit within the more general context of the overall programme and it is likely that trainees will have an educational supervisor who is responsible for their overall progress, either for the full two-year programme or for each year of the programme. So it may be that some educational appraisal may be delivered by an overall educational supervisor for the year, whilst other elements may be delivered by a trainer on the clinical team to whom the trainee is attached.

There seems little doubt that more time for both trainees and trainers will be spent on the business of appraisal and of course, yet more time still will be spent on the assessments which form such an important part of the Foundation programme. One of the principles of the Foundation years is that trainees are themselves responsible for organizing the appraisal and assessment elements of their programme and for gathering the records of this activity. This will be quite a considerable task and it will form a significant part of the trainee's life.

# What should an assessment contain?

Foundation trainees will have a number of conversations with their educational supervisor (or supervisors). These conversations need to deal with a whole range of issues. Only some of them come within a strict definition of the term 'educational appraisal' but most of them are essential for the smooth progress of an individual's training.

- Setting of educational objectives for the whole programme or at least for the whole of each year of the programme. This obviously takes place at the beginning of the year. However, a lesser version of the same process will take place at the beginning of each attachment.
- Review of progress and performance against these objectives – the second stage of appraisal. Each attachment will need at least three appraisal interviews. The first sets objectives, the second and third monitor the achievement of those objectives.
- Setting of special short- or medium-term objectives to remedy any perceived problems. (This does not necessarily mean problems with a trainee's performance; it is more likely to happen when a trainee has not had the opportunity to experience a particular service activity which is important to their own career objectives.) As people's career plans develop so it may be necessary to vary objectives and set new ones. This can take place at any stage after the start of a programme. In a few cases it will be necessary to vary or change objectives because trainees are in difficulty and they may need more focused training experience.
- Feedback on clinical performance. The single most useful thing any trainer can do is to give their trainee clear feedback upon their clinical performance. There is ample evidence that this is one of the most useful ways of supporting and accelerating learning.
- Career discussion and advice. Career support is one of the pillars of the new Foundation year programmes. Unfortunately, as things stand at the moment, the future shape of specialist training seems very uncertain, so it is very hard for a career advisor to give much advice. Nevertheless, a good system of career advice within a hospital depends upon the discussion of future career plans being part of the routine appraisal of trainees.
- Evaluation. Evaluation concerns the attachments themselves and the overall programme. Although it is a different process from appraisal, it is very helpful to trainers to receive feedback on their programme directly from trainees. Few trainers will have the time to set up a special and separate interview to do this.

# The appraisal process

There are many variants on the appraisal process but in general it breaks into three parts.

## Setting objectives

The important thing in this part of the process is that the appraiser and the appraisee should agree what is expected in the next part of the course. This goes by all sorts of names: setting objectives or goals, making an educational plan, agreeing learning objectives, etc. If possible, it is also valuable to set indicators of performance. In the Foundation years the successful completion of the assessment programme is one obvious indicator, but there might be others.

It is self-evident that the objective-setting meeting needs to happen at the start of any particular attachment in order to be of any value.

## Performance review

Once objectives have been set, subsequent meetings have a simple agenda: to agree whether or not the objectives have been met.

## Changes in objectives and unmet objectives

If objectives are to be reviewed, it follows that they may not have been met or possibly that, in retrospect, it is seen that one or other objective might not have been appropriate. The third part of the process concerns making any changes in objectives that may be appropriate and agreeing ways in which appropriate unmet objectives might be met.

# A final note on competency-based training

One of the watchwords for the proposed modernized medical careers of the future is that they will be 'competency based'. This approach regards the finished product – a trained specialist or GP – as a summation of appropriate competencies. If all the competencies are in place and have been tested, we are invited to take the view that the doctor who has competed this training is indeed competent.

There is in fact little evidence to support this approach to life. In the first place, competent and complete clinicians are exercising a huge range of different skills during their working day and it is unlikely that truly discriminatory testing is available to test all of them. Second, and more importantly, the real test of the overall skills of clinicians occurs when they are facing the unexpected and dealing with problems outside their experience to date. Such events are an inextricable part of medical life and the 'competency' which is involved is that of 'ability to deal with circumstances which at the moment we cannot quite define'. Although it is possible to think of methods of assessment that might provide a surrogate for testing for this competency, it is hard to be confident in the robustness of any such method.

The reality is that a competent professional is actually displaying an integrated mixture of skills and knowledge and any overall judgement of their competence needs to be based on a consideration of the integrated whole. Training a competent and complete professional appears to be based upon experience which is allowed to increase in range as time goes on. As the experience of the professional trainee increases, so it is possible to increase their degree of responsibility. It is obviously helpful for trainees to receive feedback on their overall performance during this process and this is probably one of the most important formative processes in the creation of a competent and complete professional.

Assessment of competencies has a perfectly valid place in training, therefore, and we can think of all sorts of skills that people need in particular specialties. There is nothing against testing these skills and it is a valuable thing to do provided that it does not consume too much resource which would be better devoted elsewhere. However, it is very important for trainees and trainers alike to understand that a sheet with all the competency boxes ticked only shows that the trainee has some of what it needs to be a competent clinician in their chosen field. There is much more besides . . .

# Reference

1. Department of Health, Social Services and Public Safety, Scottish Executive, Welsh Assembly Government. *Modernizing Medical Careers – The Next Steps. The Future Shape of Foundation, Specialist and General Practice Training Programmes*. London: Department of Health, 2003.

# 7 Assessment methods

Vijay Hajela

Trainees starting their Foundation programmes in August 2005 will have to produce evidence showing that they are competent in key areas of medical practice before they can progress to specialty training in August 2007. This evidence will be gathered through a series of work-based assessments. The four assessment methods will be: direct observation of procedural skills, mini clinical evaluation exercises, multisource feedback and case-based discussions. If all of these assessments and subsequent appraisals take place as planned then trainees could receive an unprecedented amount of high-quality, one-to-one feedback. However, organizational difficulties within trusts and delays in setting up of national systems to help collate results threaten the smooth introduction of this assessment process.

## Introduction

In order to successfully complete Foundation training, a trainee will need to produce evidence showing that they have acquired certain generic skills and that they are competent in key areas of medical practice. This evidence will be obtained through a series of work-based assessments (i.e. the assessments take place at work as opposed to going off-site to sit an exam). The emphasis will be on assessment of a trainee's performance in a variety of clinical settings as opposed to traditional knowledge-based assessments, such as written exams.[1]

## Who will be assessed?

Foundation pilots have largely concentrated on the assessment of F2 trainees. However, it is now clear that the assessment process will apply to both the F1 and F2 years. Some deaneries may feel that trusts are not quite ready for assessment of F1 trainees by August 2005 and it may be August 2006 before the first round of compulsory assessments is introduced.

In order to gain full registration, F1 trainees will need to demonstrate competence in areas outlined in the GMC's *New Doctor*.[2] However, deaneries may feel that the local arrangements currently in place for assessing PRHOs are sufficient for the August 2005–6 cohort of F1 trainees. Beyond August 2006, it is likely that both F1 and F2 trainees will need to participate in the new system of competency-based assessment. The assessment methods and process will be very similar for F1 and F2 trainees although the absolute content of what is assessed and the standards expected will obviously differ.

## What will be assessed?

Basically, the generic skills that every doctor should acquire before progressing to specialist training. These generic skills fall into key areas of practice that have been derived from the General Medical Council's document *Good Medical Practice*.[3]

- Good clinical care: especially the management of acutely sick patients, clinical decision making, awareness of limitations and utilization of clinical resources.
- Relationships with patients: in particular, good communication skills.
- Working with colleagues: written and verbal communication with colleagues and the ability to work effectively in a team.
- Good time management and the ability to prioritize work.
- Legal and ethical dimensions to practice.
- Effectiveness in teaching and training colleagues.

## What assessment methods will be used?

Four methods of assessment will be used to try and gauge a trainee's performance. A brief summary of each is given below but they are discussed in more detail later in the chapter. The absolute number of assessments expected in the F1 year is not yet clear but it will probably be fewer than the figures quoted below for the F2 year.

- *Direct observation of procedural skills (DOPS): six in the F2 year.* Assessment of basic procedures such as cannulation, giving IV medication, inserting a urethral catheter, etc. Marked by an expert, using a structured checklist.

- *Mini clinical evaluation exercise (mini-CEX: six in the F2 year*. Also known as an observed clinical encounter, this is like a clinical short case but with immediate feedback.
- *Case-based discussion (CbD)*: *6–8 in the F2 year*. A structured discussion of clinical cases managed by the trainee using their own entries into clinical notes as the basis for discussion.
- *Multisource feedback (mini-PAT: Peer Assessment Tool): 16 raters in the F2 year*. The anonymized views of numerous work colleagues (raters) are collated and fed back to the trainee at their next appraisal.

## Key issues about assessments

The assessments that take place in the Foundation programme will include the following factors.

### Trainee led

It will be the trainee's responsibility to find an appropriate person to supervise each assessment. They agree the time and location of each assessment with their supervisor as well as selecting a suitable patient or set of notes to be used in the assessment. It will also be the trainee's responsibility to ensure that all their assessments are completed before the end of their F2 year. The ultimate sanction for failure to complete the assessment process is that the trainee would not be signed off for Satisfactory Completion of Foundation Training (by the regulatory body PMETB). Without this, trainees may be unable to progress to specialty training.

### Portfolio based

Trainees will need to keep a record of their assessments in a portfolio. Throughout the year this portfolio will accumulate a body of evidence about a trainee's performance. The portfolio will provide a starting point for discussion in a trainee's subsequent appraisals.

### Used to aid trainee development

Each assessment provides the opportunity for constructive feedback of the trainee's strengths and weaknesses. By the end of each assessment at least one action should be agreed upon to help the trainee to improve their skills, knowledge or performance (e.g. to read up a certain topic or to observe a senior colleague performing a procedure). Many trainees who have undergone F2 assessments as part of F2 pilot programmes in London have commented that they found the assessments surprisingly valuable because of the feedback that they generated about their performance.

## What happens to the results of these assessments?

As already mentioned, trainees will get feedback from their supervisor straight after each assessment (excluding multisource feedback). Each trainee's educational supervisor will be responsible for reviewing the results of the assessments with the trainee at their next appraisal. The outcome of these appraisals should be an agreed 'personalized development plan' – basically suggested ways in which the trainee can work on their weaknesses and consolidate their strengths. However, it will take serious analysis to tease out all the information that these assessments can provide about performance in specific domains of practice. This is particularly true for the multisource feedback, which would be very labour intensive to analyse manually. Centralized analysis of assessments (in particular for multisource feedback) is promised and will be needed.

Systems do exist, such as for the Sheffield mini-PAT tool, that are capable of producing an overall summary of an individual's performance in each domain of practice and comparing this to their peer group (they collate all the scores and feedback about a trainee's communication skills and compare this information to the rest of the trainees in that programme. The trainee and their supervisor can then see if this is an area in which the trainee is doing well or if it needs working on). Unfortunately, a centralized data analysis system and the infrastructure capable of coping with assessments from all of the UK's Foundation trainees is not yet available. Until then each deanery will need to make local arrangements for the collation of these data and it is uncertain how this is going to work. Deaneries will be responsible for recommending satisfactory completion of Foundation training based on a summary of each trainee's assessments but it is unclear what support will be available to help produce these summaries.

## Specific issues relating to the assessment process

### Documentation

In the early days of the Foundation programme it is probable that assessments will be recorded manually on standard forms. Several copies will need to be made (one for each trainee and their educational supervisor and possibly one to be sent into the deanery or any national database). Standard forms have not yet been made available and for August 2005 each deanery may need to make their own arrangements. Electronic systems for recording assessments are under development. These will allow trainees to compile their portfolio electronically and to populate it with the results of each assessment. This will obviate the need for the endless paper records which may cause logistical difficulties initially.

## Marking assessments

It is likely that a six-point scale will be used to rate a trainee's performance in each assessment, with a score of 4 indicating the standard expected at completion of F2 training. Since this is a new year of training there remains some uncertainty about what this standard should be. Scores of 5 or 6 indicate that the trainee's performance in that domain of practice is above expectation and scores of 1 and 2 below expectation, with 3 being borderline. It is to be expected that many trainees will score less than 4 early on in their Foundation programme. This should not be regarded as failure but rather should be highlighted as an area in which further development is required. Only if a further round of assessments later in the year shows that the trainee has not improved in this same area should concern be raised.

## Time required to complete assessments (see Table 7.1)

The estimated time commitment for these assessments is likely to be considerable for both trainees and their supervisors. In total, over the year a

TABLE 7.1   Estimated assessment time per F2 trainee per year (once trainees and supervisors are familiar with the assessment process)

| Tool | Estimated time taken per assessment for supervisor (minutes) | Number of assessments per year | Total direct contact time per year (minutes) |
|---|---|---|---|
| Mini-PAT | 6 | 16 | Not applicable |
| Mini-CEX | 20 | 6 | 120 |
| DOPS | 15 | 6 | 90 |
| CbD | 20 | 6 | 120 |
| Total time | | | 5 h 30 min |

figure of 5.5 hours has been suggested. This is likely to be a minimum and until everyone becomes familiar with the assessment methodology, it may well be double this. However, a range of healthcare professionals can be enlisted to supervise the assessments; for example, for DOPS you could enlist senior nursing staff, phlebotomists or other technicians, SpRs, pharmacists and any other suitably skilled healthcare professionals. For multisource feedback, the wider the professional spread, the better. However, in many departments it may be that the only person able to perform case-based discussions or mini-CEXs is the trainee's own consultant. For hard-pressed consultants this may seem like an unwelcome extra burden at first. It will take familiarity with the assessment methods and greater confidence that the whole process is of benefit (to both the trainees and the service) for this to change.

Despite this, if all the assessments and appraisals take place as planned, trainees should receive an unprecedented amount of feedback on their performance and trusts will have more information than ever before about the competence of their most junior doctors.

## Administration

Until an electronic record of assessments is available, each hospital will need to have a system for dealing with the paperwork generated by these assessments. Copies of the results need to be sent to the trainee's educational supervisor and also to the deanery (or possibly a national assessment co-ordinating centre). This is just one role for a Foundation Programme Administrator, a vital appointment for any new Foundation programme.

## Assessors, educational supervisors and feedback

Specific training in assessment methods and in how to give feedback will be mandatory for all assessors of Foundation trainees. This will require a certain investment of time and money by trusts. Different assessors are suggested for each CbD and mini-CEX. This may prove difficult to achieve initially as it is unlikely that there will be sufficient numbers of trained assessors within each trust in the first couple of years of the Foundation programme.

Each Foundation trainee will also require a named educational supervisor. They will be responsible for ensuring that trainees understand and engage in the assessment process, and conducting regular appraisals with their trainees. At these appraisals the trainee's portfolio will be reviewed. Results from completed assessments will be discussed and areas where the trainee has performed well should be highlighted as well as those areas that require further development. A plan for futher development is then agreed upon to help the trainee to focus on specific areas in the next few months.

## What constitutes 'failure'?

One of the anticipated benefits of the new assessment process is that it will allow failing trainees to be identified earlier. A failing trainee may be flagged up by:

- an unwillingness or failure to participate in the assessment process
- failure to show improvement in areas of poor performance
- involvement in complaints, clinical incidents
- concerns raised by their educational or clinical supervisors.

At present it is not clear what will happen to poorly performing trainees who fail to complete Foundation training to the satisfaction of the new regulatory body (the Postgraduate Medical Education and Training Board – PMETB). Their deanery may recommend remedial training but the arrangements for this are not yet known.

It is also unclear what the sanctions will be for a trainee who is known by their clinical supervisors to be competent but who does not have the evidence from assessments to prove it. Initially there may be a period of grace in which to complete these assessments. But in the future it is likely that evidence of satisfactory completion of competency-based assessments will be mandatory for progression to the next stage of training.

# Assessment methods

## Case-based discussion (CbD)

What is it?

This is basically a structured discussion of clinical cases managed by the trainee. The trainee's own entries into clinical notes are the basis for the discussion. Case-based discussion is widely used in the US where it is known as chart-stimulated recall. This process provides an opportunity for trainees to explain why they acted as they did and for them to get good-quality feedback from a senior clinician. It also allows the ethical and legal framework of practice to be explored. Feedback from some London F2 pilot trainees has been very positive, some saying that it is the first time that they have had regular, structured feedback from a senior clinician.

What is involved?

The assessor selects one set of clinical notes from several in which the trainee has written. The trainee's entries form the basis for discussion about aspects of their performance. The focus of the discussion may be agreed in advance, e.g. clinical decision making, discharge planning, the ethical basis for decisions or even the accuracy of notekeeping. The discussion should include constructive feedback and end with an agreed summary of any learning points. The scoring sheet is marked with the trainee present and at least one action point is agreed upon, e.g. to start writing problem lists on each patient or to have a senior colleague check the next few discharge summaries before they are sent.

Who can supervise CbDs?

The trainee chooses the assessor although in practice, this will probably need to be a senior doctor, e.g. their supervising consultant, or GP. The process is more robust if a different assessor is chosen for each CbD but this may not be practical initially if insufficient supervisors are trained.

How long does each CbD take?

Approximately 20 minutes though this depends upon how the discussion goes and how much time the supervisor and trainee can spare.

How many are required each year?

Each trainee will probably have to complete six CbDs per year.

## Direct observation of procedural skills (DOPS)

What is it?

The trainee is observed performing a clinical procedure by someone who has substantial expertise in that particular procedure.

What is involved?

The trainee chooses the timing, the observer and the procedure to be assessed. The procedures are chosen from a standard list outlined in the Foundation curriculum. They include very basic medical procedures such as cannulation, administration of IV, IM and subcutaneous injections, insertion of a urethral catheter, obtaining arterial blood gases, etc. However, many trainees will want to have other more complex skills observed in addition to these and this will be encouraged.

The assessment of DOPS is not only concerned with the eventual outcome, e.g. did the trainee get the cannula into the vein? Things that will be marked include adequate preparation of equipment, explanation to the patient of what is about to happen, adherence to aseptic technique when appropriate, safe use of analgesia, clearing up of sharps, overall technical ability and seeking assistance when appropriate.

Who can supervise DOPS?

Anyone who is regarded as having sufficient expertise to train someone well in that procedure. For example, a senior phlebotomist may be a more suitable observer of cannulation skills than a consultant who has not cannulated a patient in years. ECG technicians, senior nursing staff, resuscitation officers, senior physiotherapists and SpRs can all be recruited to help out with this form of assessment. A different observer is suggested for each DOPS (i.e. a trainee should not get the same SpR to observe all their DOPS).

How long does each DOPS take?

This is highly dependent on the procedure but anywhere from 10 to 30 minutes.

How many are required each year?

Uncertain but between four and six per year as a minimum.

*Mini clinical evaluation exercise (mini-CEX; pronounced 'mini-keks' and not 'mini-sex'!)*

What is it?

This is a 15–20 minute snapshot of a doctor–patient relationship in which a trainee is observed taking a history or examining a patient. Essentially this is like a traditional clinical short case but with immediate feedback. Data from the US have shown that mini-CEX is reliable, valid and acceptable to trainees and clinical supervisors.

What is involved?

The trainee agrees with their supervisor an appropriate time, location and patient for the assessment. They are observed performing the task, e.g. taking a history, taking consent or examining a patient (or a combination of these). The trainee's performance is discussed at the end and their strengths and suggested areas for development are fed back. At least one action point is agreed at the end of the assessment (e.g. to read up causes and management of pleural effusions). The mark sheet is then filled in with the trainee.

Who can supervise a mini-CEX?

This will probably need to be a senior clinician (e.g. consultant/senior SpR or GP trainer). It is recommended that a different observer be used for each mini-CEX.

How long does each mini-CEX take?

Approximately 15 minutes for the clinical encounter but anywhere from 5 to 15 minutes for feedback, i.e. a total of 20–30 minutes.

How many are required each year?

Each trainee will probably have to complete six mini-CEXs per year.

## Multisource feedback (mini-PAT: Peer Assessment Tool)

What is it?

Basically multisource feedback is a way of collecting the opinions of a range of people who work with a trainee about how the trainee has performed during that post. It is also known as 360° assessment. It is likely that this tool will eventually become part of the appraisal process for all doctors from F1 to consultant.

What is involved?

F2 trainees will need to identify work colleagues whom they feel will give honest feedback about them. This may be consultants or GPs, SpRs, nursing staff, allied healthcare professionals such as pharmacists, physiotherapists, dieticians, technicians or even ward clerks. Trainees will be encourage to get feedback from a wide range of people that they work with and in particular they will be discouraged from selecting all doctors (i.e. all their friends!) If this is suspected, they may be asked to repeat the exercise.

The trainee then compiles a list of names and contact details of colleagues who have agreed to participate in the feedback process. The trainee sends this list to their F2 co-ordinator who arranges for each person to be sent a mini-PAT feedback form. Once completed, this form is returned either to a central database or the Foundation co-ordinator. An efficient administration system is required to send nominated individuals the mini-PAT forms and to chase up and collate their responses. It is anticipated that this will eventually be done centrally with the results being summarized, compared to a trainee's peer group and then being sent back to the trainee and their educational supervisor for discussion at the next appraisal. Until centralized analysis systems are up and running, this work may need to be done by the Foundation co-ordinator in each hospital.

Is the feedback anonymous?

Yes, the results are anonymized although contributors of free-text comments will need to be aware that a trainee reading their comments may be able to pick up clues from what is written.

What does giving feedback using the mini-PAT involve?

It simply involves filling in one form which takes about five minutes to complete. The form has 15 questions and a global rating scale. There is also the opportunity for free-text comments. Each of the 15 questions has a six-point scale and an 'unable to comment' option.

How many people does a trainee need to ask for feedback?

Sixteen in the first eight months of the year. In $3 \times 4$ month jobs, a trainee will need to identify eight individuals by the end of the first four months and a further eight by the end of the second four-month placement. In six-month placements, at least eight will need to be identified by the end of the first post and a further eight by halfway through the second post.

## Conclusion

Two things will be required to bring about an environment in which these assessments fit routinely into the working day. First, the confidence of trainees and supervisors that these assessments will deliver what they promise. Second, a culture change within trusts with regard to the training needs of their most junior doctors.

# References

1. Academy of Medical Royal Colleges and MMC Implementation Groups of the Department of Health, Scottish Executive and Welsh Assembly. *Curriculum for the Foundation Years in Postgraduate Education and Training*. London: Department of Health, 2005.
2. General Medical Council. *Good Medical Practice*. London: General Medical Council, 2001.
3. General Medical Council. *The New Doctor*. London: General Medical Council, 2005.

# Useful websites

*www.mmc.nhs.uk* Modernizing Medical Careers
*www.londondeanery.ac.uk* London Deanery
*www.gmc-uk.org* General Medical Council

# 8 Writing a curriculum vitae

**Ashis Banerjee**

A curriculum vitae (CV) must be fit for purpose; that is, it must help you secure your desired job. Given the importance of this document, it is often striking how little care appears to have been taken in its production. From the short-listing panel's perspective there is often little to choose between the numerous almost identical CVs that tend to be submitted for Senior House Officer positions. While the process of writing a CV is not an exact science and some variation is inevitable, some points need to be emphasized.

A CV is often mistaken by the applicant for a biographical document within which everything achieved in a relatively short life has to be enumerated and padded out in the form of a 10-page document, duly bound and indexed. The longer a CV, and also the more popular the post you have applied for, the less likely it is to be read through and the more likely it is to be discarded prematurely. The biggest problem with a long CV is that it might actually serve to bury the really important details. The real purpose of the CV is to make the readers want to meet the writer and possibly to employ her or him after an interview, and this should be achieved with the minimum number of words possible.

The purpose of the following discussion is to allow you to write a succinct CV designed to make an impression. However, nothing can guarantee you that job interview as other factors such as the nature of the competition and the nature of the personal specification vary! Do run your CV past as many senior or middle-grade colleagues as possible – they may often have useful pointers which may be potentially beneficial. Many brains put together are usually better than your own acting in isolation.

A short covering letter of application is usually all that is necessary. In hospital applications this letter is often not read and may not even be presented to the short-listing panel. The considerable variability in the content of CVs has led to increasing numbers of hospitals using application forms in the interests of equal opportunities for employment. However, a supplementary CV is often still useful.

---

**Box 8.1 Things not to include in a CV**

- Details of all schools attended, including GCSEs and A levels, numbers and grades
- Failures or negative things about yourself: failed examinations, unsuccessful projects
- Spelling mistakes
- Poor grammar
- Handwritten alterations, amendments and additions
- Lies
- Written testimonials

---

# Curriculum vitae writing

The appearance of the CV is guided by some basic rules. Plain black ink should be employed. A legible font, such as Times New Roman, Arial or Century Gothic, should be used, with a font size of 12pt being optimal. One should avoid fancy or multiple fonts. Some fonts are, in fact, more difficult to read as well as irritating to the eye. Upper-case letters and underlining should be used sparingly. The use of bold characters to emphasize key themes is helpful and breaks up the monotony of the text. Italics are best avoided. In general, the document should be photocopier and scanner friendly.

There should be generous spacing between lines but there is no need for full double spacing. A wide left-hand margin allows short-listing committee members to write notes if required. Fancy patterns and borders should be avoided. The document should be printed on good-quality bright white or cream A4 size paper, preferably 100 gram weight. Tinted paper is sometimes used but best avoided.

A frontispiece with name and qualifications and the title of post or rotation for which you are applying is helpful. Remember that applications can get misplaced and find themselves in the wrong pile for short-listing. This probably happens more often than is admitted!

The pages should be numbered. A header or footer with the name of the applicant on it is helpful for longer documents. Avoid an index; this is rather presumptuous and unnecessarily lengthens the document, making it more unwieldy. Consider binding with a slide binder rather than stapling the pages together which makes detaching them individually rather difficult. Do not send poor-quality photocopies, which suggest a multiple mailing exercise! The document should not be folded and should be sent in an A4 envelope.

Long sentences and long chunks of text should be avoided. The use of bullets for subsections or lists helps to break up the text into more manageable segments which are more friendly on the eye. Poor spelling and grammar should be eliminated, as they indicate a poor knowledge of the English language and thereby may suggest poor comprehension of the spoken word and poor communication skills in general. The use of a spell-checker is not enough, as these do not recognize many medical words and may not understand the context in which particular words are used. Abbreviations should generally not be used. There should not be any repetitions of textual material.

The second page contains important personal details. It starts with full name, address, contact details (phone, fax and e-mail), date of birth (day, month and year), sex (not always obvious from one's name!), nationality/residency status and current post. Marital status, maiden name, number and ages of children/dependants are optional and probably not necessary. Religious and political affiliation should not be declared; there is always someone who will disapprove! Early childhood details, while of nostalgic value, should be avoided. Photographs, often provided by Teutonic applicants in particular, are only required for professions where being photogenic is in itself a qualification! Include details of licence to practise: eligible for limited/full. If already registered with the GMC, please provide the GMC number.

---

**Box 8.2 CV structure**

- Frontispiece
- Personal details
- Qualifications (awards/prizes)
- Current post
- Career interests
- Previous posts
- Publications and presentations
- General interests

---

Qualifications should be listed in reverse chronological order along with grades achieved where relevant (for example, first class honours for a degree) and awarding institutions. The subjects of any thesis submitted must be documented where applicable. A section for prizes and awards can be provided separately or incorporated in the qualifications system to avoid the short-lister to have to move to-and-fro in the document. You may include a section for any additional roles carried out which indicate administrative and interpersonal skills, e.g. treasurer of a club, education representative at medical school, entertainment officer for the mess.

Junior doctors are better placed to submit chronological CVs as opposed to functional CVs, for those with long work histories and frequent job changes. Previous posts held are listed in reverse chronological order and should include title of job, name of institution, name of lead or supervising consultants worked for. It is important to include objective data, i.e. facts and figures, relating to workload (numbers of patients, hours worked, frequency of on-call commitments), types of patients treated and special interests within the department. If the CV is long, it may be useful to merely list the appointments and to provide a separate section on clinical experience which summarizes the experience gained from different positions. Clinical experience implies abilities and responsibilities and procedures which you are competent to perform, if certified or validated. Merely providing long lists of non-validated competencies is of no benefit whatsoever in helping short-listing. It is necessary to emphasize special skills gained from each position held.

Non-clinical experience includes teaching (formal and informal; grades of staff taught such as nurses, undergraduate or postgraduate medical students, other healthcare professionals), audit, management, research, computing skills (databases, packages, programs). A knowledge of foreign languages may be useful to include.

Any gaps in employment must be accounted for, even if this involved undertaking a period of travel or some other recreational interest.

Publications and presentations are enumerated in a separate section, in chronological order. If greater than five in number in each section, it is preferable to separate these into presentations, publications, letters and books. Publications include abstracts, original papers, editorials or leaders, reviews, book chapters, letters (state if original contribution) and miscellaneous. List publications in the Vancouver style, including names of all authors, full title, title of journal, year, volume and page numbers.

Audit experience usually should be mentioned. This should include title of audit, where and when performed, and what the outcome was. Involvement in audit that involved deficiencies in the service that were then addressed and led to improvements is often a major selling point.

Relevant courses and meetings attended should be listed, including dates and venues.

Information technology skills should be identified and outlined, listing software packages in which you are proficient.

The career intentions and interests section is very important but often missing from CVs. A career plan, emphasizing your knowledge of and interest in the specialty or job chosen, is very valuable. This should incorporate an approximate time schedule for short-term and intermediate- to long-term career objectives.

General interests should be listed, as they can give an idea of the total individual. These should be classified as recreational, sporting, cultural and political. This section should not be too extensive, as it might prompt questions about whether there will be any time left for work commitments! Any national or international achievements and awards should be emphasized.

Referees' names, including e-mail addresses, should be provided. It is important to obtain their permission beforehand. It is not necessary to include these in the body of CV, in order to reduce the size of the document and to cut down on photocopying costs.

The CV should be updated regularly as and when things occur. This makes for a hassle-free process in the production of a document for the next position being applied for.

A portfolio should be kept in addition, including logbook, copies of published papers, summaries or handouts from presentations and audits, letters of praise or thanks. It is possible that in the near future these will be inspected at the time of interview and they certainly are important in the process of revalidation.

It is important to allow for postal delays and delays in the hospital internal mail system. Late submissions are often seen as evidence of being sloppy and disorganized.

---

### Box 8.3    Elements of a good CV

- Concise
- Appealing visual layout
- Organized information

---

# Experiences of a Foundation year 2, Senior House Officer

Louise Ma

Modernizing Medical Careers has finally hit us with a bang. As you know, this long-planned overhaul of the medical training system has two main objectives: first, to give us doctors a more structured training programme post medical school, and second, perhaps more importantly, to allow the public to have a more standardized and formalized framework on which their doctors can be judged and assessed. Many inside and outside the profession have debated the relative merits or otherwise of the idea of Modernizing Medical Careers (MMC), as well as its actual implementation. That debate I leave to others. The purpose of this chapter is to provide a practical example experience under the Foundation year 2 (FY2) pilot scheme which I hope will prove helpful to those of you who will need to navigate the same waters.

Under MMC what came out for us junior doctors was the Foundation programme (the 'programme').[1] In short, the programme is two years of 'general training which forms the bridge between medical school, and specialist/general practising training. It will comprise a series of placements in a variety of specialties and healthcare settings. Learning objectives for each stage will be specific and focused on demonstration of clinical competencies'.[1] All very well but what does it actually mean for those of us going through it?

## Finding the job

I was nearing the middle of my second house post and it was time to start looking for a Senior House Officer position. I started via the well-known channels, such as bulletin boards and websites (e.g. *www.bmjcareers.com*, *www.doctors.net.uk*) and came across the usual medical rotations, i.e. stand-alone six-month posts or two-year rotations. I then noticed the jobs for the FY2 programme which were described as building upon the knowledge, skills and attributes developed in the Pre-Registration House Officer year. 'The FY2 will encompass the generic competencies applicable to all areas of medicine, including team working, the use of evidence and data, time management, communication and IT skills, although the main focus of training will be the assessment and management of the acutely ill patient.'

Since I had always wanted to explore my options in the specialties before pursuing what will ultimately be a career in medicine, but found the postings on offer too rigid to accommodate that desire, the FY2 premise caught my interest immediately. FY2 would allow me to have one year of training (where the actual day-to-day duties were not too dissimilar to other Senior House Officer positions, except that many clinical practices would need to be assessed) in which rotation amongst several specialties of my choice (e.g. accident and emergency, obstetrics and gynaecology, paediatrics, ear, nose and throat, orthopaedics, medicine and surgery, etc.) was possible.

FY2 was therefore especially appealing to me, and should be for any graduate like myself who wants to achieve a broader specialty experience before choosing a particular career pathway. Since the year of training is either divided into six months in A&E and then two three-month positions in other areas, or equally into four three-month positions in different areas, gone is the unrealistic pressure often placed on junior doctors to make a crucial career decision without the full benefit of practical experience and informed judgement.

## Getting the job

Most of the written applications for programme jobs required details on personal clinical experience, knowledge and skills. Of particular interest to selectors appeared to be house officers who have displayed an interest in

TABLE 9.1 Example of rotations

| August | December/February | April/May |
| --- | --- | --- |
| A&E | COE | Medicine |
| A&E | Medicine | Paediatrics |
| A&E | ENT | COE |
| A&E | Orthopaedics | Surgery |
| A&E | Obstetrics & gynaecology | Paediatrics |
| A&E | COE | Orthopaedics |
| A&E | Surgery | Paediatric surgery |
| A&E | Medicine | Intensive care unit |
| A&E | Medicine | Psychiatry |

Derived from Lewisham University Hospital Trust, Homerton University Hospital Trust and Barking, Havering and Redbridge Hospitals NHS Trust evidence-based medicine, and especially those who can show evidence of keeping up to date with medical knowledge and practices. There were then the usual leadership and teamwork questions, e.g. examples of both during clinical incidents.

Once the written application had been accepted, there were then the interviews. Given that the programme was still being introduced, I attended two interviews for the FY2 pilot programme. Each interview comprised a panel of three consultants from different specialties, lasting 20 minutes each. Lines of questioning mainly surrounded previous medical experience, as well as more personal curriculum vitae aspects such as reasons for selecting the FY2 pilot scheme, future plans and motivation. Given my stated interests, there was also a lengthy discussion on management of an acutely ill patient with an ethical dilemma. There was one question that did catch a few candidates out, which was to give an example of a mistake I made in the past and what I learned from it.

I found that the consultants were generally supportive of candidates' goals and were very flexible in terms of structuring the one-year programme. I ended up spending the year doing accident and emergency; care of the elderly and general medicine – which was my first-choice rotation schedule.

## Starting the job

Like the first day at any new hospital, there was the usual full-day induction – vast amounts of information handed out and equally voluminous amounts of paperwork to be filled in. Trainees were introduced to the main programme supervisors, who welcomed us to the new pilot scheme and explained that although the London Deanery and other Royal Colleges had not yet recognized these as training posts, we would be getting more training than the average Senior House Officer, with an extra hour of teaching a week and other extra courses. I had specifically checked with the Education Officer at my previous hospital and the advice I received was that it would only be a matter of time before the paperwork was finalized and therefore the jobs being recognized as training approved (as I write this now, the FY2 Programme will be backdated as a training post upon completion).

Amongst all the bits and pieces that we were given was the course curriculum, i.e. the core skills and knowledge that must be attained by the end of the year. They include:

- management of acutely ill patients
- resuscitation and do not resuscitate orders

- management of patients while 'on take' with the team
- discharge planning
- making appropriate investigations and interpretation of those results
- competence of core practical procedures (i.e. venepuncture, injections).

A more detailed curriculum can be found on the NHS website.[2]

## Doing the job

### Courses and teaching

Once a week, an extra hour was set for teaching. As trainees came from differing backgrounds and specialties, the teaching topics had to be made relevant to all our tasks, both professional and personal. Examples were 'Interpreting arterial blood gas results', 'Making good use of the radiology department', 'Good medical practice', etc. A particularly useful teaching session was interview technique. Trainees were asked to bring their own CV for the interviewers and, like real job interviews, questions that would frequently feature were fired at us in a 'mock' setting. We were given an opportunity to perform under pressure and receive constructive criticism in an area of our training which is crucial but often neglected.

Whilst we were encouraged to attend many extra training sessions that were relevant (e.g. advanced life support courses on offer), three extra courses were especially designed for the programme trainees, all of which enabled us to become more well-rounded medical professionals.

- *Communication*: a whole day of role plays with actor-patients, going through scenarios such as breaking bad news and encounters with an angry patient/relative, etc.
- *Pharmacology*: raising awareness of common prescription mistakes, and the workings of the pharmacy department.
- *HELP (How to Evaluate and treat Life-threatening Problems)*: aimed at trainees who had not done advanced life support/trauma life support. This highlighted ways to identify acutely ill patients with respiratory, circulatory or neurological problems and how to immediately manage them.

### Taster week

To further broaden our experiences in other specialties, a 'taster week' was devised. This consisted of going to work in another department, to get 'a taste' of that particular area. These were extremely useful and in my particular experience, we were given the choices of microbiology/clinical biochemistry/ haematology or oncology.

## General practice sessions

One hour a week, each trainee had to attend a morning session with a local general practice. This is another way for the NHS to expose more doctors to general practice, as nearly half of the trainees ultimately choose this specialty as a career. For those undecided, this was great first-hand experience with primary care. For others who were already set on other specialties, being fully involved in these sessions gave a greater insight into what happens after hospital patients are discharged. One particularly memorable occasion for me was finding a recently discharged stroke patient attending the general practice for a check-up. It made me realize how critical a good working relationship between primary care and hospitals is for the good of the patient.

# Assessments

In line with the stated aim of the programme (i.e. focus on a more formalized definition of quality), four key assessment tools are used:

1. mini-PAT (peer assessment tool)
2. mini-CEX (clinical evaluation exercise)
3. DOPS (directly observed procedural skills)
4. CbD (case-based discussions).

## Mini-PAT

This is a 360° evaluation of the trainee by eight healthcare professionals in order to generate feedback from a range of co-workers across the domains of *Good Medical Practice*.[3] Any doctor, nurse or allied healthcare professional can be nominated by the trainee. The questionnaire asks for feedback on clinical care, medical practice, relationships with patients and colleagues, etc. A sample of the assessment tool can be found at *www.mmc.nhs.uk/ assessment_miniPAT.asp?m=4*.

## Mini-CEX

This is a 'snapshot' of a doctor–patient encounter, be it in the wards, general practice or hospital outpatient clinics. The assessments lasts for 15–20 minutes, with the following areas taken into account:

- history taking
- clinical examination skills
- professionalism
- clinical judgement
- communication skills
- organization/efficiency
- overall clinical care.

An evaluation (lasting around five minutes) then takes place with a Senior Specialist Registrar, staff grade, consultant or general practitioner in which the background and complexity of the case are discussed and further improvements suggested. Figure 9.1 shows the evaluation sheet.

## DOPS

This is a practical skill assessment tool in which any Senior Registrar, consultant, nurse or allied healthcare professional who is trained in any of the following practical skills can be the assessor.

| | |
|---|---|
| Venepuncture | Taking an ECG |
| Cannulation | Airway care |
| Blood cultures (peripheral, central) | Nasogastric tube insertion |
| Intravenous infusion | Urethral catheterization |
| Injections (IM, IV, intradermal, subcutaneous) | Arterial blood gas sampling<br>Others |

Although many of these skills would have been assessed before at earlier points of any medical training, the DOPS ensures that there is consistency of performance regardless of the trainee's background. Moreover, the 'Others' section allows more complicated procedures to be assessed, such as insertion of a chest drain or performing an appendectomy. Figure 9.2 shows a DOPS evaluation sheet.

## CbD

This is the assessment of documentation, presentation and management of particular patients where the trainee has made significant clinical decisions on the patient's management. Only Specialist Registrars, staff grades, consultants or general practitioners can be assessors. This type of evaluation has been practised since the 1980s in the USA where it is called 'chart-stimulated recall'.[4] The areas to be appraised are:

- medical record keeping
- clinical assessment

Please complete the questions using a cross: ☒    Please use black ink and CAPITAL LETTERS

| Doctor's | Surname | |
|---|---|---|
| | Forename | |

GMC Number: [ ][ ][ ][ ][ ][ ][ ]    **GMC NUMBER MUST BE COMPLETED**

| Clinical setting: | A&E ☐ | OPD ☐ | In-patient ☐ | Acute Admission ☐ | GP Surgery ☐ |
|---|---|---|---|---|---|

| Clinical problem category: | Airway ☐ | Breathing ☐ | Circulatory ☐ | Neuro ☐ | Psych/Behav ☐ | Pain ☐ |
|---|---|---|---|---|---|---|

| New or FU: | New ☐ | FU ☐ | Focus of clinical encounter: | History ☐ | Diagnosis ☐ | Management ☐ | Explanation ☐ |
|---|---|---|---|---|---|---|---|

| Number of times patient seen before by trainee: | 0 ☐ | 1-4 ☐ | 5-9 ☐ | >10 ☐ |
|---|---|---|---|---|

| Complexity of case: | Low ☐ | Average ☐ | High ☐ | Assessor's position: | Consultant ☐ | SASG ☐ | SpR ☐ | GP ☐ |
|---|---|---|---|---|---|---|---|---|

| Number of previous mini-CEXs observed by assessor with any trainee: | 0 ☐ | 1 ☐ | 2 ☐ | 3 ☐ | 4 ☐ | 5-9 ☐ | >9 ☐ |
|---|---|---|---|---|---|---|---|

| Please grade the following areas using the scale below: | Below expectations for F2 completion | | Borderline for F2 completion | Meets expectations for F2 completion | Above expectations for F2 completion | | U/C* |
|---|---|---|---|---|---|---|---|
| | 1 | 2 | 3 | 4 | 5 | 6 | |
| 1  History Taking | ☐ | ☐ | ☐ | ☐ | ☐ | ☐ | ☐ |
| 2  Physical Examination Skills | ☐ | ☐ | ☐ | ☐ | ☐ | ☐ | ☐ |
| 3  Communication Skills | ☐ | ☐ | ☐ | ☐ | ☐ | ☐ | ☐ |
| 4  Clinical judgement | ☐ | ☐ | ☐ | ☐ | ☐ | ☐ | ☐ |
| 5  Professionalism | ☐ | ☐ | ☐ | ☐ | ☐ | ☐ | ☐ |
| 6  Organisation/Efficiency | ☐ | ☐ | ☐ | ☐ | ☐ | ☐ | ☐ |
| 7  Overall clinical care | ☐ | ☐ | ☐ | ☐ | ☐ | ☐ | ☐ |

*U/C Please mark this if you have not observed the behaviour and therefore feel unable to comment.

**Anything especially good?**     **Suggestions for development**

**Agreed action:**

| | Not at all | | | | | | | | | Highly |
|---|---|---|---|---|---|---|---|---|---|---|
| Trainee satisfaction with mini-CEX | 1 ☐ | 2 ☐ | 3 ☐ | 4 ☐ | 5 ☐ | 6 ☐ | 7 ☐ | 8 ☐ | 9 ☐ | 10 ☐ |
| Assessor satisfaction with mini-CEX | 1 ☐ | 2 ☐ | 3 ☐ | 4 ☐ | 5 ☐ | 6 ☐ | 7 ☐ | 8 ☐ | 9 ☐ | 10 ☐ |

Have you had training in the use of this assessment tool?: ☐ No   ☐ Yes: Face-to-Face   Time taken for observation: (in minutes) [ ][ ]
☐ Yes: Written Training   ☐ Yes: Web/CD rom

Assessor's Signature:     Date: [ ][ ] / [ ][ ] / [0][5]     Time taken for feedback: (in minutes) [ ][ ]

Assessor's Surname: [ ][ ][ ][ ][ ][ ][ ][ ][ ][ ][ ][ ][ ][ ][ ][ ][ ][ ][ ][ ][ ][ ][ ][ ]     0399259883

FIGURE 9.1  Mini-Clinical Evaluation Exercise (CEX)

| | | |
|---|---|---|
| Please complete the questions using a cross: ☒ | | Please use black ink and CAPITAL LETTERS |

Doctor's     Surname

Forename

GMC Number:      **GMC NUMBER MUST BE COMPLETED**

Clinical setting:

| A&E | OPD | In-patient | Acute Admission | GP Surgery |
|---|---|---|---|---|
| ☐ | ☐ | ☐ | ☐ | ☐ |

Procedure Number:
(Please see guidance)     In other please specify:

Assessor's position:

| Consultant | SASG | SpR | GP | Nurse | Other |
|---|---|---|---|---|---|
| ☐ | ☐ | ☐ | ☐ | ☐ | ☐ |

Number of previous DOPS observed by assessor with any trainee:

| 0 | 1 | 2 | 3 | 4 | 5-9 | >9 |
|---|---|---|---|---|---|---|
| ☐ | ☐ | ☐ | ☐ | ☐ | ☐ | ☐ |

Number of times procedure performed by trainee:

| 0 | 1-4 | 5-9 | >10 |
|---|---|---|---|
| ☐ | ☐ | ☐ | ☐ |

Difficulty of procedure:

| Low | Average | High |
|---|---|---|
| ☐ | ☐ | ☐ |

| Please grade the following areas using the scale below: | Below expectations for F2 completion | | Borderline for F2 completion | Meets expectations for F2 completion | Above expectations for F2 completion | | U/C* |
|---|---|---|---|---|---|---|---|
| | 1 | 2 | 3 | 4 | 5 | 6 | |
| 1 Demonstrates understanding of indications, relevant anatomy, technique of procedure | ☐ | ☐ | ☐ | ☐ | ☐ | ☐ | ☐ |
| 2 Obtains informed consent | ☐ | ☐ | ☐ | ☐ | ☐ | ☐ | ☐ |
| 3 Demonstrates appropriate preparation pre-procedure | ☐ | ☐ | ☐ | ☐ | ☐ | ☐ | ☐ |
| 4 Appropriate analgesia or safe sedation | ☐ | ☐ | ☐ | ☐ | ☐ | ☐ | ☐ |
| 5 Technical ability | ☐ | ☐ | ☐ | ☐ | ☐ | ☐ | ☐ |
| 6 Aseptic technique | ☐ | ☐ | ☐ | ☐ | ☐ | ☐ | ☐ |
| 7 Seeks help where appropriate | ☐ | ☐ | ☐ | ☐ | ☐ | ☐ | ☐ |
| 8 Post procedure management | ☐ | ☐ | ☐ | ☐ | ☐ | ☐ | ☐ |
| 9 Communication skills | ☐ | ☐ | ☐ | ☐ | ☐ | ☐ | ☐ |
| 10 Consideration of patient/professionalism | ☐ | ☐ | ☐ | ☐ | ☐ | ☐ | ☐ |
| 11 Overall ability to perform procedure | ☐ | ☐ | ☐ | ☐ | ☐ | ☐ | ☐ |

*U/C Please mark this if you have not observed the behaviour and therefore feel unable to comment.

**Please use this space to record areas of strength or any suggestions for development.**

| | Not at all | | | | | | | | | Highly |
|---|---|---|---|---|---|---|---|---|---|---|
| Trainee satisfaction with DOPS | 1 ☐ | 2 ☐ | 3 ☐ | 4 ☐ | 5 ☐ | 6 ☐ | 7 ☐ | 8 ☐ | 9 ☐ | 10 ☐ |
| Assessor satisfaction with DOPS | 1 ☐ | 2 ☐ | 3 ☐ | 4 ☐ | 5 ☐ | 6 ☐ | 7 ☐ | 8 ☐ | 9 ☐ | 10 ☐ |

Have you had training in the use of this assessment tool?:

☐ No    ☐ Yes: Face-to-Face    ☐ Yes: Written Training    ☐ Yes: Web/CD rom

Time taken for observation: (in minutes)

Assessor's Signature:     Date: ☐☐ / ☐☐ / 0 5

Time taken for feedback: (in minutes)

Assessor's Surname:

7339084453

FIGURE 9.2   Direct Observation of Procedural Skills (DOPS)

- investigation and referrals
- treatment
- follow-up and future planning
- professionalism
- overall clinical care.

The whole assessment lasts no longer than 20 minutes and provides a great tool for trainees to keep track of their own progress. During a 'post-take' ward round, the whole medical team is often so engaged that the finer details or personal appraisals of junior doctor clerking are ignored. The CbD is an opportunity for trainees to make sure their work is assessed, outside the busy ward environment and in a more constructive manner. Figure 9.3 shows the CbD evaluation form.

## Summary

In addition to providing the general public with a more definable quality guarantee, these assessment tools are also a big plus to junior doctors since they formalize performance review in a more transferable manner. There are structured, official evaluations from clinical skills to good medical practice, where more than one trainer takes part in the appraisals. Gone are the days when a consultant's appraisal was a quick comment on passing in a corridor or a brief chat in the office. Moreover, these assessments will be recognized and can be accumulated as evidence for future job applications. This gives a junior doctor confidence and proof that they can perform up to and beyond the standard level of their grade.

# Appraisals

Similar to most Senior House Officer posts, there are three meetings with the educational supervisor throughout the programme. The initial meeting is to plan the year so that the trainee is given the right opportunities and support to reach their learning objectives. The second and third meetings are to ensure that the trainee is on track with these learning objectives, and to try and resolve any problems encountered along the way.

In addition, there are programme appraisals of the core curriculum. Progress is logged mid-year and then again at the end of the programme. The benefit of this appraisal is that an overall picture can be made of the whole year's progress. If a trainee has had particular problems with certain assessments,

Please complete the questions using a cross: ☒    Please use black ink and CAPITAL LETTERS

Doctor's    Surname

Forename

GMC Number:    **GMC NUMBER MUST BE COMPLETED**

Clinical setting:    A&E ☐    OPD ☐    In-patient ☐    Acute Admission ☐    GP Surgery ☐

Clinical problem category:    Airway ☐    Breathing ☐    Circulatory ☐    Neuro ☐    Psych/Behav ☐    Pain ☐

Focus of clinical encounter:    Medical Record Keeping ☐    Clinical Assessment ☐    Management ☐    Professionalism ☐

Complexity of case:    Low ☐    Average ☐    High ☐    Assessor's position:    Consultant ☐    SASG ☐    SpR ☐    GP ☐

| Please grade the following areas using the scale below: | Below expectations for F2 completion | Borderline for F2 completion | Meets expectations for F2 completion | Above expectations for F2 completion | | U/C* |
|---|---|---|---|---|---|---|
| | 1 | 2 | 3 | 4 | 5 | 6 | |
| 1  Medical record keeping | ☐ | ☐ | ☐ | ☐ | ☐ | ☐ | ☐ |
| 2  Clinical assessment | ☐ | ☐ | ☐ | ☐ | ☐ | ☐ | ☐ |
| 3  Investigation and referrals | ☐ | ☐ | ☐ | ☐ | ☐ | ☐ | ☐ |
| 4  Treatment | ☐ | ☐ | ☐ | ☐ | ☐ | ☐ | ☐ |
| 5  Follow-up and future planning | ☐ | ☐ | ☐ | ☐ | ☐ | ☐ | ☐ |
| 6  Professionalism | ☐ | ☐ | ☐ | ☐ | ☐ | ☐ | ☐ |
| 7  Overall clinical judgement | ☐ | ☐ | ☐ | ☐ | ☐ | ☐ | ☐ |

*U/C Please mark this if you have not observed the behaviour and therefore feel unable to comment.

**Anything especially good?**    **Suggestions for development**

**Agreed action:**

Trainee satisfaction with CbD    Not at all  1 ☐    2 ☐    3 ☐    4 ☐    5 ☐    6 ☐    7 ☐    8 ☐    9 ☐    Highly 10 ☐

Assessor satisfaction with CbD    1 ☐    2 ☐    3 ☐    4 ☐    5 ☐    6 ☐    7 ☐    8 ☐    9 ☐    10 ☐

Have you had training in the use of this assessment tool?:    ☐ No    ☐ Yes: Face-to-Face    ☐ Yes: Written Training    ☐ Yes: Web/CD rom    Time taken for observation: (in minutes)

Assessor's Signature:    Date: ☐☐ / ☐☐ / 0 5    Time taken for feedback: (in minutes)

Assessor's Surname:    1058310042

**FIGURE 9.3**  Case-based Discussion (CbD)

these would be noted and passed on to the overall programme supervisor, so that they could be rectified before the trainee finishes the post.

## Conclusion

Given the pilot nature of the programme during my participation, there were a few teething problems, e.g. some of the teaching sessions and practical skills would be more appropriate for F1 trainees than F2, which will undoubtedly be resolved when the programme becomes compulsory in the year 2006.

The FY2 programme has been set up to help junior doctors bridge the gap between Pre-Registration House Officer and their future career, by building up their clinical skills and knowledge for the effective management of acutely ill patients in a hospital setting. It allows doctors who are yet unsure of their chosen career to have a taster of different specialties before committing to a life-long career in a particular field. With the advent of the new European Working Time Directive,[5] fewer working hours means a much more structured approach to teaching is vital, to ensure junior doctors are trained adequately for the demands made of them. From my own experience, the FY2 scheme seems to be shaping up to the task nicely.

### Acknowledgements

To Professor Shelley Heard, Dean of Postgraduate Medicine at the London Department of Postgraduate Medical and Dental Education, and to Dr Julian C Archer, Medical Education Research Fellow from the National Foundation Assessment Programme Medical Education Research Office, for providing the sample assessment tools for publication.

## References

1. Modernizing Medical Careers: About the Foundation Programme. *www.mmc.nhs.uk/foundation.asp?m=3*
2. Academy of Medical Royal Colleges and MMC Implementation Groups of the Department of Health, Scottish Executive and Welsh Assembly. *Curriculum for the Foundation Years in Postgraduate Education and Training*. London: Department of Health, 2005.
3. General Medical Council. *Good Medical Practice*. London: General Medical Council, 2001.
4. Maatsch JL. Assessment of clinical competence on the Emergency Medicine Specialty Certification Examination: the validity of examiner ratings of simulated clinical encounters. *Ann Emerg Med* 1981; **10**: 504–7.

5. Department of Health. European Working Time Directive.*www.dh.gov.uk/PolicyAndGuidance/ HumanResourcesAndTraining/ WorkingDifferently/EuropeanWorkingTimeDirective/fs/en.*

# Useful websites

*www.dh.gov.uk/PolicyAndGuidance/HumanResourcesAndTraining/Working Differently/EuropeanWorkingTimeDirective/fs/en* European Working Time Directive
*www.gmc-uk.org/index.htm* General Medical Council
*www.mmc.nhs.uk/index.asp?m=1* Modernizing Medical Careers

# 10 Junior doctors' hours

**Giles Walker**

Assigning work patterns to junior doctors has never been more complicated than at present. Currently the hours worked by junior doctors are governed by two sets of rules: the existing rules of the New Deal and the more recent European Working Time Directive (EWTD) rules. Although the EWTD is seen as having superseded the New Deal, the New Deal rules must still be followed. In addition, it must be remembered that pay banding is based solely on New Deal criteria. EWTD rules are based on Health and Safety legislation whereas the New Deal is employment legislation.

## The New Deal

The New Deal for junior doctors was introduced in 1991, to provide limits for the average weekly hours worked. Upper limits were set on both average contracted hours per week (the time a doctor is required to be available) and the average actual hours per week (the time a doctor is considered to be working). Rest guidelines were also introduced, to avoid the situation where junior doctors were working for two or three days with little rest, to protect patient safety. Different types of rota were considered to demand different amounts of time worked, from full-shift rotas (100% of time worked, contracted hours equal to actual hours) to on-call rotas (50% of out-of-hours time worked). In practice, this distinction often did not reflect reality and no distinction was made between juniors who were on site when on call and those whose on-call was carried out from home. Under the old system for calculating additional pay for out-of-hours work, additional duty hours (ADHs) therefore frequently did not reflect work intensity.

Subsequently, the current system of pay banding was introduced, based on total hours worked and the proportion of those hours which were unsocial (7 pm to 8 am and weekends).

The rest requirements outlined in the New Deal give rise to two figures for the hours of any rota. The 'contracted hours' is defined as the average weekly time that the doctor is on duty, including rest periods during partial shifts and on-calls. The 'actual hours' is defined as the time spent working and excludes rest periods. Different shift types are assumed to have different amounts of rest time; the actual hours are limited to 56 hours per week in all cases but the contracted hours can be higher, depending on the type of shifts worked in the rota.

## Types of shift

### Full shift

Full shifts are considered to apply when the doctor is working all the time during a duty period, apart from natural breaks and 30 minutes' rest after four hours' continuous duty. These shifts are limited to 14 hours duration. For purposes of calculating hours, the contracted hours and actual hours (i.e. the hours engaged in work) are considered to be the same. The minimum time off between shifts is eight hours.

### Partial shift

Partial shifts are considered to apply when a part of the duty period can be taken as rest. In this case there should be a reasonable expectation that 25% of the out-of-hours part of the duty period will be available for rest. The term 'reasonable expectation' is taken to mean that this will be the case in 75% or more of the shifts. Partial shifts can be up to 16 hours long, in which case up to four hours of that duty period will be rest. These slightly longer shifts can be used to provide out-of-hours cover while all others in the rota will be working normal working days. Partial shift rotas allow a maximum contracted 64 hours per week, which gives a maximum actual hours of 56 per week. Since these rotas tend to be residential, the maximum contracted time will be governed by EWTD requirements.

### Twenty-four hour partial shift

This pattern again implies a reasonable expectation that 25% of the duty period will be taken as rest (i.e. six hours). In addition to this, the rest in this case must include a four-hour continuous break from work between 10 pm and 8 am. It is also specified that where a doctor is expected to work after this four-hour break, a maximum of four hours can be worked before the end of the shift; in practice, this means that 24-hour partial shifts tend to begin and end at 1 pm at the latest. Twenty-four hours' rest is required after a 24-hour partial shift. Again, the maximum contracted duty is limited to 64 hours per week but will in reality be lower due to EWTD requirements.

### On-call shift

On-call shifts assume a reasonable expectation that 50% of the out-of-hours time is available for rest (i.e. eight hours in a 24-hour shift with a normal working day of eight hours, 12 hours out of 24 hours at weekends). The doctor can continue on to a normal working day following the on-call, allowing a maximum duty period of 32 hours or 56 hours at weekends). The maximum contracted duty is limited to 72 hours per week, again giving a maximum actual time worked of 56 hours per week. The on-call can be carried out either in the hospital or at home but the former is less common now as these hours all count towards the EWTD maximum limit.

### Hybrid rotas

Different shift types can be utilized in constructing a rota. This may be required due to the different requirements of weekend days, where all of the contracted hours are subject to rest requirements. Weekdays include a normal working day which is treated as a full shift, reducing the amount of rest needed. This was most obvious with on-call rotas where 50% of weekend hours were required to be taken as rest; substituting partial shifts at these times will then allow a lower rest requirement. The contracted weekly hours limit will depend on the proportion of types of shift used in the rota, while the maximum actual hours per week will remain at 56.

## Prospective cover

The majority of rotas require that duties which occur during annual or study leave taken by a doctor are covered by another doctor on the rota, so that all duties on a rota are covered internally. This avoids reliance on finding locum cover in these situations, which can be difficult to provide reliably. Where this occurs, it must be remembered that this practice will increase the average number of hours worked each week and must be included in calculations to determine both the legality and the pay banding for any rota.

## Pay banding

In December 2001 the current system for calculating pay was introduced. The basic salary of junior doctors was supplemented by a multiplier determined by the total hours worked and the proportion of those that were unsocial. Broadly speaking, doctors who work between 40 and 48 hours per week will be in band 1 and doctors who work between 48 and 56 hours per week will be in band 2. Within these pay bands are divisions dependent on the proportion of those hours which are unsocial, with band A attracting the highest multiplier for the most out-of-hours work.

At the introduction of pay banding, the highest multiplier was band 3. This pay band was paid to those working a rota which was outside the maximum hours limit. This band no longer exists as rotas with actual hours above 56 per week are illegal and can no longer be used.

The pay bands in use at present are allocated as follows.

### Band 2A

- Between 48 and 56 average hours worked per week
- Most antisocial hours – for shift-based rotas where more than one-third of hours are out of hours (7 pm to 8 am) or work one weekend in three or more; on-call rotas working one in six or more or one in three weekends or more and fulfilling Criteria R (see note below)
- Multiplier is 1.8 (i.e. total pay will be the basic salary multiplied by 1.8)

### Band 2B

- Between 48 and 56 average hours worked per week
- Least antisocial hours – for shift-based rotas, less than one-third of hours are out of hours or less than one weekend in three; on-call rotas which do not fulfil Criteria R
- Multiplier is 1.5

### Band 1A

- Between 40 and 48 average hours worked per week
- Most antisocial hours – for shift-based rotas, more than one-third of hours out of hours or more than one in four weekends worked; on-call rotas working one in six or more; on-call rotas working one in eight or more or one in four weekends or more and fulfilling Criteria R
- Multiplier is 1.5

### Band 1B

- Between 40 and 48 average hours worked per week

- Moderate antisocial hours – shift rotas not fulfilling criteria for band 1A; on-call rotas not fulfilling criteria for band 1A but working one in eight or less frequently and resident for clinical or contractual reasons
- Multiplier is 1.4

Band 1C

- Between 40 and 48 average hours worked per week
- On-call rotas working one in eight or less frequently and not resident for clinical or contractual reasons
- Multiplier is 1.2

Notes

- Prospective cover must be taken into account when determining the frequency of on-calls or weekends worked
- Criteria R applies when a junior doctor is resident and carrying out work after 7 pm or is non-resident but carries out more than four hours work after 7 pm on 50% or more occasions

Flexible trainees who work less than 40 hours per week on average are categorized into bands FA (most antisocial hours), FB (least antisocial hours) and FC (all hours worked between 8 am and 7 pm on week days). Those in bands FA and FB receive the full basic salary supplemented by the appropriate multiplier (FA 1.25, FB 1.05); those in band FC are paid pro rata based on the full basic salary being paid for 40 hours per week (i.e. a flexible trainee who works 30 hours per week will receive 75% of the basic salary).

# European Working Time Directive

## Background

In September 1990 the Draft Directive on Organization of Working Time was drawn up after initial talks in Strasbourg. In November 1993 the Directive was accepted by the European Council of Ministers, for implementation on 23 November 1996. This Directive stipulated a 48-hour working week. The United Kingdom secured a number of concessions at that time; a seven-year 'grace' period was allowed, so that the Directive would be implemented in November 2003. During this time a number of groups of workers were exempt from the Directive: transport workers (air, rail, road, sea and inland waterway workers), police and junior doctors. Implementation of the Directive for junior doctors was on 1 August 2004. In addition, a phased implementation of the maximum hours was allowed: the hours limit introduced in 2004 was 58, with a reduction to 56 hours per week in 2007 and finally to 48 hours per week in 2009.

Rest guidelines also had to be implemented from 2004, principally 11 hours uninterrupted rest in any 24-hour period. Derogation from the Directive was allowed, so that where less than 11 hours rest was given between shifts, compensatory rest could be given to redress this. Twenty-four hours continuous rest during a one-week period or 48 hours continuous rest during a two-week period was also stipulated, but similar requirements were already in place from the New Deal rules.

The European Working Time Directive is based on Health and Safety law rather than employment law and consequently, compensatory rest has been taken to mean unpaid rest purely to ensure that the worker is adequately rested to continue working safely. However, the interpretation of this part of the EWTD remains the least clear area of the rules.

Since the New Deal rules already stipulated a maximum average working week of less than 56 hours, the EWTD was initially not thought to pose a problem. The hours above this, for example up to 16 additional contracted hours per week in on-call rotas, were to be rest time and would therefore not interfere with the EWTD requirements. Problems would be encountered with the rest requirements but changes to rotas together with derogation would allow compliance with the Directive.

However, this view changed in October 2000, when a case heard by the European Court of Justice produced a ruling on the interpretation of rest which differed from the view in use in the UK.

## The SiMAP and Jaeger rulings

The Sindicato de Medicos de Asistencia Publica (SiMAP) was a group of doctors from Valencia who contended that the time they spent on call at work should not be considered as rest. The European Court of Justice ruled in their favour, on the basis that time spent in the place of work was too restrictive to be considered as rest.

> 'Time spent on call by doctors... must be regarded in its entirety as working time... if they are required to be present at the health centre'
> (European Court, October 2000)

The SiMAP ruling was upheld in the European Court in 2003 in the case of Landeshauptstadt Kiel v. Norbert Jaeger (the Jaeger ruling).

> 'On-call duty performed in a place determined by the employer constitutes in its totality working time even where the doctor is permitted to rest at his place of work when his services are not required.' (European Court, September 2003)

These rulings meant that all time spent in the hospital while on duty, which includes time spent resting or even sleeping, must be considered as work as far as EWTD implementation was concerned.

Consequently resident on-call rotas, which were allowing up to 72 hours per week in the hospital, had to be considered in their entirety (i.e. the contracted hours, not the actual hours) as time worked. In this case, on-call rotas had to be reduced to be compliant and this has led to the need for much greater change than was previously expected. Resident on-call rotas became undesirable generally, so that partial- and full-shift rotas have become prevalent.

## Compensatory rest

Compensatory rest under the EWTD applies to time off between shifts, rather than rest time during shifts under the New Deal rules, except in the case of an on-call from home. Essentially, if the 11 hours uninterrupted rest is either not given between shifts or is interrupted by work, in the case of a non-resident on-call, this rest must be compensated.

In addition to confirming the SiMAP ruling, the Jaeger ruling also stated that compensatory rest should be given before the start of the subsequent shift (i.e. within 24 hours).

The exact interpretation of compensatory rest has been disputed since the EWTD rules came out. One perspective states that if a rest period is less than 11 hours for any reason, the whole rest period must be repaid with an extra full 11-hour rest period. It has also been contended that this compensatory rest should be paid rest, giving rise to the possibility of a doctor who is disturbed for a short period having to take a full day and a half off in compensation.

Another perspective on this is that the compensatory rest should be equivalent to the loss of rest; for example, a rota which provides 10 hours' rest between two shifts must then provide 12 hours' rest after the second shift. This ensures that the doctor is adequately rested before starting the next duty period, which is the purpose of EWTD. In addition, this perspective holds that the compensatory rest does not have to be paid, since the EWTD is aimed at providing adequate rest rather than a change to pay. At present, the latter perspective is more widely supported, but could be challenged at any point in the European Court.

## Effects of EWTD

To continue to provide 24-hour cover in hospitals, required for acute specialties, a number of options have been available. The simplest answer, to staff rotas with more doctors to give EWTD-compliant rotas, is both expensive and also often impractical.

One of the problems with implementing the EWTD rules has been to continue to provide sufficient training for junior doctors. Employing a large number of doctors to fill a rota may then lead to dilution of training opportunities during the normal working week. In practice, a small increase in the number of doctors working many rotas was needed to maintain the number of doctors available during the working week to both fulfil service commitments and allow training, since in general doctors were having to go home after a night shift where they had previously worked the following day.

In addition to this, some cases required a reduction in the number of doctors working out of hours; this particularly applies to some smaller subspecialties, where a small number of junior doctors had worked a resident on-call rota primarily to provide ward cover. This situation applies most obviously in larger (often teaching) hospitals with a number of tertiary referral services. In some of these cases a number of specialties may merge rotas to provide one rota to cross-cover all specialties, reducing the number of doctors on call and the number of hours for each doctor.

Another important point to come out of the work done prior to the implementation of EWTD is that a substantial proportion of work done by junior doctors out of hours is unnecessary. This work fell into a number of categories: clinical work which could be done by another healthcare professional, clerical work, duplicative work (repeat clerking when reviewing a patient) and routine work which should be carried out during the normal working day. This has prompted the introduction of nurse practitioners and clinical technicians in a number of hospitals, to take on some of the out-of-hours workload, and systems to avoid unnecessary work being left to the out-of-hours team; overall, the aim has been to reduce the workload in line with the reduction in junior doctor numbers.

Another important effect of EWTD implementation that has been noticed by many junior doctors is reduction in pay banding in many jobs. Up to now this has been an effect of reducing hours and pay to allow for an increase in numbers of junior doctors without incurring high costs. Without a change in the SiMAP and Jaeger rulings, this trend is likely to continue to its logical conclusion in 2009; at that point all rotas will have to be under 48 hours per week, implying that band 1 will become the maximum available pay band.

The changes in working patterns towards full-shift rotas and the associated changes in working practice towards generic skill training to allow greater cross-cover between subspecialties are also likely to continue as the 2009 deadline for 48-hour average working weeks approaches.

# 11 | Professional and Linguistic Assessment Board Test (PLAB)

**Simon Edward**

The Professional and Linguistic Assessment Board tests are conducted by the General Medical Council (GMC) to test the skills and ability of overseas doctors coming from outside the European Union to practise medicine in the UK under supervised posts in the National Health Service (NHS).

Initially, both professional and linguistic capabilities of the candidates were assessed through a single examination conducted in the UK at the same time. It has since evolved into a multiphase assessment (though it has continued to carry the same name) with the linguistic component being tested separately.

A candidate has to first obtain a certified competence in the use of the English language through the IELTS exam (International English Language Testing System) conducted by the British Council, IDP Education Australia or the University of Cambridge. It is mandatory for a candidate to obtain a minimum score in the IELTS to gain eligibility to sit for the PLAB exam.

The professional component is assessed in two parts:

- PLAB part 1 conducted periodically in the UK and overseas centres all over the world
- PLAB part 2 conducted throughout the year at the GMC office in London.

## IELTS

The IELTS is conducted on a weekly basis in over 120 countries, testing the listening, reading, writing and speaking skills of the candidate. It tests the general English proficiency of the candidate in their ability to work in an English-speaking country like the UK. A candidate has to have an overall band score of 7.0 in the academic module (with a minimum score of 7.0 in the speaking task and a minimum of 6.0 in the others) to be eligible to sit for the PLAB part 1 exam. It is valid for a period of two years before which the candidate needs to take the PLAB part 1 exam. In the unfortunate event of the candidate being unable to obtain the required scores, the exam can be taken again only after a minimum period of 90 days.

The evaluation has been quite strict and therefore adequate preparation is warranted. Material for preparations is widely available and it is advisable to prepare for the exam with material produced according to the Cambridge English Speakers of Other Languages (ESOL)'s question paper production cycle. For further assistance, many IELTS test centres and language schools offer IELTS preparation courses that can be quite helpful though not necessary for all candidates.

The test fee charged per candidate is £88 and the application form and further details can be obtained from the official website *www.ielts.org*. Of late, the British Council has been conducting briefing sessions for candidates on the day prior to the exam.

# PLAB part 1

PLAB part 1 is conducted in the UK and various overseas centres once in every 2–3 months. There is no limit to the number of attempts allowed.

The emphasis of the exam is on clinical management and includes science as applied to clinical problems. The exam is confined to core knowledge, skills and attitudes relating to conditions commonly seen by SHOs, to the management of life-threatening situations and to rarer, but important, problems. The exam assesses the ability to apply knowledge to the care of patients. The subject matter is defined in terms of the skill and the content.

## Eligibility requirements

To be eligible to apply for the PLAB exam, you must have:

- a primary medical qualification acceptable for limited registration. It is mandatory that the qualification must be obtained from an institution that figures in the *World Directory of Medical Schools: www.who.int/hrh/ wdms/en/*
- an adequate score in the academic module of the IELTS, as detailed above.

## Booking a place for the examination

An application for the PLAB part 1 exam can be made online or by posting an application form downloaded from the GMC website. The cost of the examination is £145. Further details can be obtained from the website: *www.gmc-uk.org*.

## Preparation

Part 1 tests the clinical knowledge of the candidate in the form of extended matching questions (EMQs) and single best answer (SBA) questions. It is a three-hour exam comprising 200 questions in total with one mark awarded for every correct answer; no marks are deducted for a wrong answer or failure to answer a question. The scoring is done through the Angoff method wherein a panel of experienced doctors decides upon a standard score that may be expected from an SHO for the particular paper and candidates are evaluated in comparison to the set standard. Therefore the pass score varies for every exam and usually, anecdotally, appears to be around 120–135. It mainly tests the candidate's skills in diagnosis, investigations and management knowledge in the context of clinical practice.

## Extended matching questions

Extended matching questions are grouped into themes. Each theme has a heading that states what the questions are about. Within each theme there are several numbered options that are listed as possible answers. Following this list of options are questions that you should answer, choosing the one most likely option. An option can be used more than once or not used at all. More than one option may seem correct but you must choose the most appropriate option.

The key to success in this exam is therefore practice but you will also benefit from reading prescribed books such as:

- *Oxford Handbook of Clinical Medicine*
- *Oxford Handbook of Clinical Specialties*
- *Clinical Medicine* (Kumar & Clark).

These books cover most of the topics that figure in the PLAB part 1 exams. Many books are available to assist with preparation for EMQs but beware of low-cost books that may not always give the correct answers to all the questions. Some suggested standard books and courses available are:

- *1000 Extended Matching Questions* by Una Coales: *www.rsmpress.co.uk*
- PASTEST series for PLAB 1 – books and online courses: *www.pastest.co.uk*
- online courses by *www.123doc.com* and *www.onexamination.com*.

You will benefit from doing as many EMQs as possible. Some themes tend to repeat in consecutive exams and there are Internet groups related to PLAB that freely offer invaluable tips in preparation and past EMQs.

Since 200 questions have to be solved within 180 minutes, time management is of the utmost importance. It is therefore advisable to skim through the entire paper within the first 10–15 minutes and eyeball the themes known to you and solve them first and then attempt the tougher ones. Inability to complete the paper has been the bane of many a failed candidate. Many candidates have noticed that many of the easy questions appeared in the latter part of the paper and were not attempted due to lack of time. Since there is no negative marking, an attempt should be made to answer all the questions.

# PLAB part 2

The PLAB part 2 exam takes place only at the GMC office in London (see end of chapter for contact details). It is conducted all through the year on Monday to Friday though there may be short periods of breaks once or twice a year.

Part 2 consists of an objective structured clinical examination (OSCE). It takes the form of 14 clinical scenarios or 'stations' as well as a rest station and a pilot station. Each station requires you to undertake a particular task. Some will involve talking to or examining the patient and some will involve demonstrating a procedure on an anatomical model, e.g. suturing a wound or giving cardiac massage to the patient (dummy). The examiner will be closely observing you doing the tasks. Each task lasts for five minutes exactly, with one minute between stations.

## Cost

The fee for taking the OSCE is currently £430 to be paid in advance. Fees sent from other countries must be in sterling bankers draft or money order and must be payable to the GMC. The fee is exclusive of bank charges.

## Applying for the exam

You may only book a place on part 2 of the test once you have passed part 1. You must pass part 2 within three years of the date you passed part 1. You may have up to four attempts at part 2 of the test and then you will need to retake PLAB parts 1 and 2 again.

Due to the large number applying for the PLAB part 2, it may take up to six months before a candidate can be allotted a place for the exam. Booking online over the GMC website is quickest and you will be able to obtain confirmation of the date immediately. For this purpose you have to write to the GMC to request a PIN number and password immediately after receiving confirmation of the booking of PLAB part 1 dates. This saves valuable time and prevents unforeseen delays in planning the journey to the UK.

## Skills tested

The main skills tested in part 2 of the test are:

- communication
- history taking
- clinical examination
- practical skills
- emergency management.

### Communication skills

Communication skills are tested through the observation of interaction between the candidate and another person, usually a simulated patient or the examiner. You are expected to know the major legal and ethical principles set out in *Duties of a Doctor* (*www.gmc-uk.org*). It is very important to gain rapport with the patient on commencing the station. It must be emphasized that each component carries some points, including greeting the examiner, greeting the patient, shaking hands, introducing oneself, ensuring confidentiality and privacy, requesting a chaperone in appropriate situations, ensuring that the patient is able to comprehend what is being discussed, listening to and empathizing with the patient's problems, social courtesy and etiquette.

Examples of communication skills tested include:

- explaining diagnosis, investigation and treatment
- involving the patient in the decision making
- checking understanding
- communicating with relatives
- communicating with healthcare professionals
- breaking bad news
- seeking informed consent/clarification for an invasive procedure or a post mortem
- dealing with anxious patients or relatives
- giving instructions on discharge
- giving advice on lifestyle, health promotion or risk factors.

## History taking

This aspect of the PLAB OSCEs tests your clinical acumen in eliciting an appropriate history from the patient based on the presentation as given in the station. Since there are only five minutes for each station, it is sometimes not possible to complete some stations. You must not be disheartened by this, as what is being tested is your approach to a patient and your ability to elicit an appropriate history in a systematic manner and not completion of history taking and arriving at a provisional diagnosis. Therefore you must not be in a hurry but ask relevant questions without interrupting the patient while he is speaking.

## Clinical examination

You will be assessed on your ability to conduct a physical examination of a standardized patient. A standardized patient is an actor who has been trained to display signs as and when required by the station. In certain circumstances, the examination will be carried out on a mannikin or model.

You are expected to be competent to carry out any basic physical examination. Examples are examination of the chest, heart, breast, hand, hip, knee and shoulder. You must be able to perform a rectal or bimanual vaginal examination. You must also be able to use the appropriate equipment in carrying out an examination of, for example, the ear or the eye.

Due to medicolegal implications, it is very important to request a chaperone in appropriate situations when a male doctor is examining a female patient. Consent needs to be obtained at every step of the examination while at the same time explaining the procedure in language that the patient is able to understand. Examination of the mental state is treated as a form of clinical examination for the purpose of this test.

You will also be marked on your ability to treat a patient with respect for their privacy and dignity and attention to their comfort. You will need to take this into account, while bearing in mind that you have only five minutes for each station.

## Practical skills

You will be assessed on your ability to perform common practical procedures, examples of which are given below.

- Taking blood pressure
- Venepuncture
- Inserting a cannula into a peripheral vein

- Giving intravenous injections
- Mixing and injecting drugs into an intravenous bag
- Giving intramuscular and subcutaneous injections
- Suturing
- Interpreting an ECG, X-rays or results of other investigations
- Bladder catheterization
- Taking a cervical smear
- Safe disposal of sharps

Emergency management

Examples of emergency management situations include dealing with postoperative collapse, acute chest pain, trauma assessment (initial and secondary), and basic adult and paediatric cardiopulmonary resuscitation. A cardiopulmonary resuscitation station is almost always present in PLAB part 2 OSCEs. It is very important to pass in the CPR station because of its importance and the significance attached to it in the practice of medicine in the UK.

## The OSCE stations

Stations are chosen from a matrix of medical areas (e.g. cardiovascular, neurological, surgical) and skill areas (e.g. history taking, practical, examination), with a view to sampling across the range of medical and skill areas. An actor, who has been provided with a detailed script beforehand, plays the patient. The examiner is supposed to observe you and not intervene, except in very limited circumstances.

You have one minute before entering the station to read the instructions, which may tell you to, for example, examine a patient, take a history and give a diagnosis or carry out a practical procedure. The instructions also give basic information about the patient, such as his or her name, age and major symptoms.

Each station has a number of sections or objectives (e.g. Communication, Past History, Diagnosis) that you do not see but which are set out on the examiner's mark sheet. The examiner awards a grade between A and E for each objective.

Each objective is weighted, with the total weightings for each station adding up to 100%. An overall grade is calculated for each station. You must obtain a 'C' grade or above in 10 or more stations to pass part 2 of the test. You cannot pass if you obtain grade E for more than one station.

Once inside the examination room, stand outside your first station booth (you will be told which is your first station) and read the candidate instructions outside the booth. You will also be asked to use an antiseptic solution prior to entering every station. You have one minute to read the instructions. Do not enter the booth until the bell rings for the start of the station.

When the bell rings, enter the booth. Inside the booth there will be an examiner. In some stations there may, in addition, be an observer. Where appropriate, there will also be a simulated patient. There will also be an additional set of candidate instructions for you to refer to, if you wish to do so. If you have been unable to read the instructions completely in the one minute while standing outside, it is most advisable to read them completely from the set provided by the examiner.

When you enter the booth, the examiner will greet you and check your name and candidate number as shown on your badge, which will be provided to you at the candidate briefing. He or she will also check that you understand the candidate instructions. Once you have started the station, do not speak to the examiner unless the candidate instructions for that station require you to do so.

It is very important to address the patient appropriately as stated in the instructions. It may be worthwhile to memorize the surname before entering the station as some past overseas candidates have found it difficult to remember them later. Carry out the task(s) required by the instructions.

Where there is a mannikin at the station, address any comments or explanations to the examiner, not to the mannikin. Where there is a simulated patient, the candidate instructions for that station will tell you whether you should address the examiner or the patient.

A bell will ring after 4.5 minutes to warn you that there are only 30 seconds remaining. Try and complete the discussion but if unable to do so, politely apologize about your lack of time and thank the patient and examiner before leaving the station. The tasks at some stations, in particular those tasks requiring practical skills, may take less than five minutes to complete. If you do finish early, remain in the booth until the five-minute bell rings.

When the five-minute bell rings, leave the station.

Your first station may be a rest station, in which case there will be no one present in the booth. Rest stations will be clearly labelled.

There will be one minute between stations. During that time, move to the next station, read the candidate instructions and wait outside the booth until the bell rings to signal the start of that station. The stations are numbered clearly from 1 to 16. Move in the direction indicated. GMC staff will always be available to assist.

## Further tips on preparation

In summary, to be able to perform well in the PLAB part 2 OSCEs, practice makes perfect. Candidates can obtain further assistance by taking courses offered in many places in the UK or by undertaking clinical observerships under a consultant in an NHS trust.

As a clinical observer, you can have hands-on experience of the practice of medicine in the UK and this will prove most helpful while preparing for the PLAB part 2 OSCE. You should approach consultants well in advance for clinical attachments and it may take 2–4 months before you are successful in obtaining one.

Some web addresses of well-known courses for PLAB part 2 are listed below:

*www.plabmaster.com*
*www.plabtutor.com*
*www.vishwamedical.com*
*www.birminghamplabcourse.com*
*www.plabtrainer.com*

These courses can cost anywhere from £150 to £400, depending on the type of course. They will allow you to practise skills where mannikins are required as most coaching centres have mannikins for candidates to practise on. They are also great places to find practice partners for the exam.

Doctors can also join network groups that give invaluable information regarding PLAB. Some popular websites are:

● *www.aippg.net*
● *www.rxpgonline.com*
● *www.bapio.co.uk.*

Taking coaching classes and attending mock exams are no doubt helpful but the most important aspect that needs to be emphasized is – practice, practice and more practice. Practice will make you more confident and allay anxiety. A group of three candidates is ideal to practise for the exam as one can keep time and play the examiner while the others can pose as candidate and patient.

After taking the PLAB part 2 exam the results will be announced on the GMC website in around two weeks' time and a letter of confirmation will reach the candidate in around three weeks' time.

After passing the PLAB part 2, you are eligible to apply for Senior House Officer jobs only if you have prior postgraduate clinical experience for a period of 12 months at an institution approved by the medical registration authorities in the appropriate country.

# Useful contact

General Medical Council
Regent's Place
350 Euston Road
London NW1 3JN
Telephone +44 (0) 845 357 3456
Fax +44 (0) 20 7915 3558
E-mail: *registrationhelp@gmc-uk.org*
Website: *www.gmc-uk.org*

# USEFUL ADDRESSES

British Council
Bridgewater House
58 Whitworth Street
Manchester M1 6BB
Tel: 0161 957 7755
*www.britishcouncil.org*

British Medical Association
BMA House
Tavistock Square
London WC1H 9JP
Tel: 020 7387 4499
*www.bma.org.uk*

Faculty of Accident & Emergency
35–43 Lincoln's Inn Fields
London WC2A 3PE
Tel: 020 7405 7071
*www.faem.org.uk*

General Medical Council
Regent's Place
350 Euston Road
London NW1 3JN
Tel: 0845 357 3456
*www.gmc-uk.org*

Immigration and Nationality
Directorate
Home Office
Lunar House
40 Wellesley Road
Croydon CR9 2BY
Tel: 0870 606 7766
*www.ind.homeoffice.gov.uk*

Medical Defence Union
230 Blackfriars Road
London SE1 8PJ
Tel: 020 7202 1500
*www.the-mdu.com*

Medical Protection Society
33 Cavendish Square
London W1G 0PS
Tel: 0845 605 4000
*www.mps.org.uk*

Postgraduate Medical Education and
Training Board
5th floor, 64 Wimpole Street
London W1G 8YS
Tel: 020 7563 6897
*www.pmetb.org.uk*

Royal College of Anaesthetists
48–49 Russell Square
London WC1B 4JY
Tel: 020 7813 1900
*www.rcoa.ac.uk*

Royal College of General
Practitioners
14 Princes Gate
London SW7 1PU
Tel: 020 7581 3232
*www.rcgp.org.uk*

Royal College of Obstetricians and
Gynaecologists
27 Sussex Place
Regent's Park
London NW1 4RG
Tel: 020 7772 6200
*www.rcog.org.uk*

Royal College of Ophthalmologists
17 Cornwall Terrace
London NW1 4QW
Tel: 020 7935 0702
*www.rcophth.ac.uk*

Royal College of Paediatrics and
Child Health
50 Hallam Street
London W1W 6DE
Tel: 020 7307 5600
*www.rcpch.ac.uk*

Royal College of Pathologists
2 Carlton House Terrace
London SW1Y 5AF
Tel: 020 7451 6700
*www.rcpath.org*

Royal College of Physicians of
Edinburgh
9 Queen Street
Edinburgh EH2 1JQ
Tel: 0131 225 7324
*www.rcpe.ac.uk*

Royal College of Physicians of
Ireland
6 Kildare Street
Dublin 2
Tel: 00 353 1 661 6677
*www.rcpi.ie*

Royal College of Physicians of
London
11 St Andrew's Place
Regent's Park
London NW1 4LE
Tel: 020 7935 1174
*www.rcplondon.ac.uk*

Royal College of Physicians and
Surgeons of Glasgow
232–242 St Vincent Street
Glasgow G2 5RJ
Tel: 0141 221 6072
*www.rcpsglasg.ac.uk*

Royal College of Psychiatrists
17 Belgrave Square
London SW1X 8PG
Tel: 020 7235 2351
*www.rcpsych.ac.uk*

Royal College of Radiologists
38 Portland Place
London W1B 1JQ
Tel: 020 7636 4432
*www.rcr.ac.uk*

Royal College of Surgeons of
Edinburgh
Nicolson Street
Edinburgh EH8 9DW
Tel: 0131 527 1600
*www.rcsed.ac.uk*

Royal College of Surgeons of
England
35–43 Lincoln's Inn Fields
London WC2A 3PE
Tel: 020 7405 3474
*www.rcseng.ac.uk*

Royal College of Surgeons in
Ireland
123 St Stephen's Green
Dublin 2
Tel: 00 353 1 402 2100
*www.rcsi.ie*

Royal Society of Medicine
1 Wimpole Street
London W1G 0AE
Tel: 020 7290 2900
*www.rsm.ac.uk*

Specialist Training Authority of the
Medical Royal Colleges
70 Wimpole Street
London W1G 8AX
Tel: 020 7935 8586
*www.sta-mrc.org.uk*

# INDEX